D0438160

DISCARD

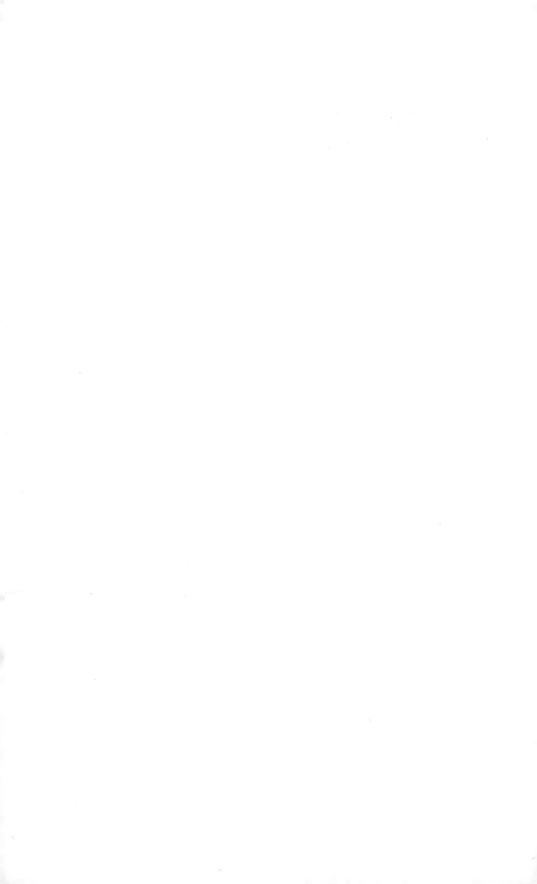

Food and Nutrition Controversies Today

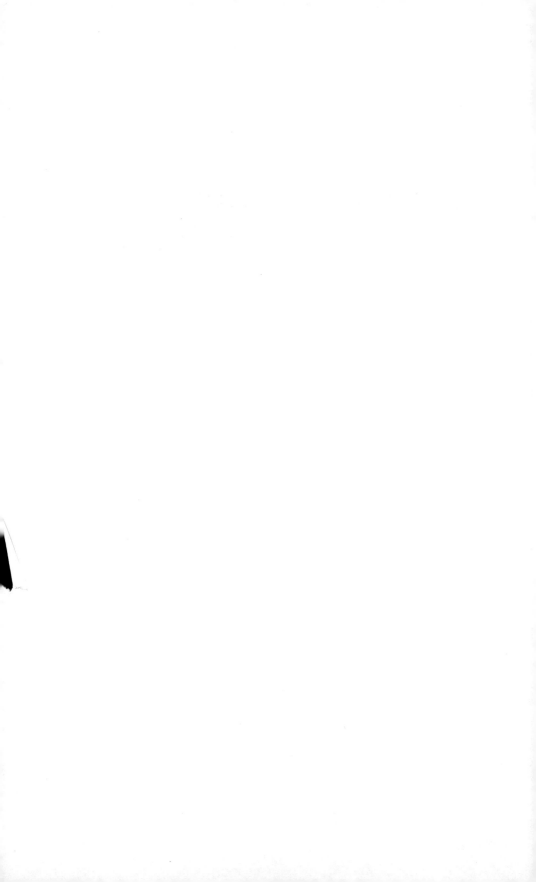

Food and Nutrition Controversies Today

A Reference Guide

**Myrna Chandler Goldstein and
Mark A. Goldstein, M.D.**

GREENWOOD PRESS
Westport, Connecticut • London

Library of Congress Cataloging-in-Publication Data

Goldstein, Myrna Chandler, 1948–
  Food and nutrition controversies today : a reference guide /
Myrna Chandler Goldstein and Mark A. Goldstein.
      p. cm.
  Includes bibliographical references and index.
  ISBN 978-0-313-35402-1 (alk. paper)
  1. Nutrition—United States. 2. Food—United States—Safety measures.
3. Food adulteration and inspection—United States. 4. Food Industry and
Trade—United States. I. Goldstein, Mark A. (Mark Allan), 1947– II. Title.
  TX357.G5745   2009
  363.19'2620973—dc22   '   2008047832

British Library Cataloguing in Publication Data is available.

Copyright © 2009 by Myrna Chandler Goldstein and Mark A. Goldstein, M.D.

All rights reserved. No portion of this book may be
reproduced, by any process or technique, without the
express written consent of the publisher.

Library of Congress Catalog Card Number: 2008047832

ISBN: 978-0-313-35402-1
First published in 2009
Greenwood Press, 88 Post Road West, Westport, CT 06881
An imprint of Greenwood Publishing Group, Inc.
www.greenwood.com

Printed in the United States of America

∞™

The paper used in this book complies with
the Permanent Paper Standard issued by the National
Information Standards Organization (Z39.48-1984).

10 9 8 7 6 5 4 3 2

We dedicate this book with love and affection to our first grandchild, Aidan Zev Goldstein, born February 8, 2008.

Contents

Acknowledgments

First and foremost, I thank Mark A. Goldstein, M.D., my husband and coauthor. Researching and writing a scholarly book is a monumental task. It is extraordinarily helpful to have someone to share ideas and to provide continuous input. Of course, like many other physicians, Mark is a superb editor, and his editorial skills proved invaluable on a number of occasions.

I also thank Vince Burns, who formerly served as Greenwood's editorial director and senior editor of Praeger and Greenwood. Without Vince, there would be no book. Very early in the process of researching and writing the book, serious problems developed. It was only because of Vince's personal intervention that these were resolved.

Finally, I thank the librarians at our local library in Lincoln, Massachusetts. Thanks to the interlibrary loan system, the librarians obtained the countless numbers of books that I required. I truly appreciate how graciously the librarians fulfilled my seemingly endless number of requests.

Introduction

It seems never ending. Society is continuously and constantly bombarded with messages about food and nutrition. The government insists that imported food is safe and carefully monitored. Yet, very little of the food is inspected, and just about everyone is aware of the periodic outbreaks of food poisoning. In a country dealing with record numbers of overweight and obese people, experts often disagree about the best ways to lose weight. Should one eat a diet that is high in protein and low in carbohydrates or one high in carbohydrates and low in protein? Or is the raw diet a better way? Is it safe? Healthful? The average consumer is at a clear disadvantage. It is not easy to sort through the options and opinions.

Although there are a myriad of food and nutrition controversies, this book has focused on just sixteen. We attempted to select the most interesting concerns, as well as those that are commonly discussed in the media. The chapters are designed to serve as introductions, presenting the various sides of the controversies. Researchers have studied each of the topics extensively. Many of them have been the subjects of books. If your interest is sparked, you may easily find additional resources to review, such as the numerous references listed at the end of each chapter. All the chapters close with listings of Websites and endnotes.

Chapter 1

Antioxidants

Antioxidants are in the news all the time. From the advertising, they appear to have a seemingly limitless number of benefits. But how much is media promotion and how much is reality?

The last time you left a half-eaten apple on the kitchen counter, it turned brown. The apple was literally attacked by free radicals, highly reactive oxygen molecules that are a by-product of normal metabolism.

Free radicals not only decay apples they also destroy living cells. As a result, they have been associated with a number of illnesses and medical problems. Most degenerative diseases, such as arthritis, cataracts, and diabetes, are linked to free radical damage. Free radicals also attack the brain and central nervous system and have been linked to heart disease and all types of cancer. In addition, they weaken the immune system in various ways.

Though free radicals are able to harm a wide variety of tissues in the body, most frequently, they hurt body fats. They injure the nucleic acid bases that form DNA and prevent the DNA from correctly duplicating itself.

As dismal as this scenario may sound, the body is not helpless. It produces enzymes that neutralize free radicals, and it uses antioxidants from foods (and sometimes supplements) to counteract the damaging effect.

Clearly, antioxidants are faced with a daunting task. In an article entitled "Anti-Aging with Antioxidants," which was published in 2000 in *Better Nutrition*, the authors note that antioxidants must work constantly to slow down the oxidation process. "These kamikaze life-saver molecules continually seek and destroy free radicals, sacrificing themselves and self-destructing to save other healthy cells from certain death."[1]

While the number of antioxidants keeps growing, careful research studies have not been conducted on all of them. Furthermore, there is

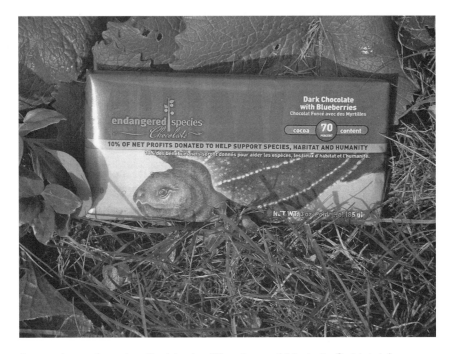

A sweet way to eat antioxidants. (Courtesy of Mark A. Goldstein)

some disagreement about correct dosages. The Food and Drug Administration (FDA) considers antioxidants to be dietary supplements or nutrient additions to the diet. As such, they are not subject to presale analysis by the FDA. Nonetheless, it is useful to review current beliefs on a few of the well-known antioxidants.

VITAMIN C

Perhaps the most recognized antioxidant is vitamin C (ascorbic acid). Although most animals synthesize their own vitamin C, primates, such as humans, do not. Therefore, all vitamin C must be obtained from the diet. According to the U.S. Department of Agriculture, some good sources of vitamin C are red sweet peppers, kiwi fruit, oranges and orange juice, grapefruit juice, strawberries, Brussels sprouts, and papaya.[2]

In the early 1970s, Linus Pauling, who won a Nobel Prize in chemistry and a second one for peace, began to champion megadoses (one to four grams per day) of vitamin C. Pauling believed that such large quantities of this antioxidant could prevent and cure colds. The medical community greeted Pauling's beliefs with skepticism. It warned that people on such high doses were at risk for serious problems such as kidney stones and vitamin B deficiency.

Despite the warnings, many people have placed themselves on high doses of vitamin C. As a rule, there have been few negative effects. Since vitamin C is a water-soluble vitamin, any excess intake is eliminated in the urine. In *Your Miracle Brain,* which was published in 2000, Jean Carper, the author, states that vitamin C appears to be very safe, even at high doses. "No toxicity has been detected at doses of 20,000 milligrams a day, the amount Dr. Linus Pauling took. You may experience loose bowel movements after taking high doses of vitamin C, but they subside when you lower the dose."[3]

There have been many studies on vitamin C supplementation. Some find it beneficial; others conclude that it neither benefits nor harms individuals; and still others find that it has a negative impact. For example, a study published in the journal *Cancer Cell* in 2007 describes how researchers gave vitamin C to mice that had been implanted with human lymphoma or prostate cancer cells. Researchers found that vitamin C did indeed inhibit the growth of some of the tumors.[4] Similarly, in a study conducted at The Institute for Medical Psychology and Behavioral Neurobiology, at the University of Tubingen, Germany, and described in a 2002 *USA Today* magazine article, researchers found that people who took two 500-milligram sustained-release vitamin C capsules four times a day for fourteen days were able to "blunt the rise in blood pressure accompanying acute psychological stress" better than those who did not take the doses of vitamin C. According to Stuart Brody, a researcher, "Blood pressure just before the stress, and up to 40 minutes after, was significantly lower in the vitamin C group."[5]

In another study published in 2007 in the *European Journal of Nutrition,* Japanese researchers examined the role that vitamin C may play in reducing the incidence of age-related cataracts in men and women between the ages of forty-five and sixty-four. After five years of study, they found that, "a higher vitamin C intake was associated with a reduced incidence of cataracts in both sexes."[6]

A study completed by researchers at the University of California, Berkeley, and published in 2004 in the *Journal of the American College of Nutrition* found that vitamin C supplements may reduce the levels of C-reactive protein in the body—"a marker for inflammation and chronic disease risk in humans." All of the 160 healthy participants were smokers or people exposed to second-hand smoke. After only two months of taking around 500 milligrams of vitamin C per day, participants "saw a 24 percent drop in plasma C-reactive protein (CRP) levels." The researchers concluded that, "Plasma CRP itself may serve as a potential target for reducing the risk of atherosclerosis, and antioxidants, including vitamin C, should be investigated further to confirm their CRP-lowering and anti-inflammatory effects."[7]

Meanwhile, a study on a number of antioxidants, including vitamin C, which was published in 2007 in the *Archives of Internal Medicine*, attempted to determine if antioxidants could play a role in the prevention of cardiovascular events, such as heart attacks and strokes, in women already at risk for these illnesses. Researchers found "no overall effects of ascorbic acid."[8] In an effort to determine if there is any evidence that vitamin C (and vitamin E) may help prevent cancer, researchers evaluated thirty-eight studies for a piece published in 2006 in the *Journal of General Internal Medicine*. They found little reason to believe that vitamin C supplements play any significant role in the prevention and/or treatment of cancer.[9]

An article that appeared in *Family Practice News* in 2000 reports on a speech given by James H. Dwyer to the American Heart Association's Fortieth Annual Conference on Cardiovascular Disease Epidemiology and Prevention. In the speech Dwyer reports that the "regular use of vitamin C supplements may accelerate, not retard, the progress of carotid atherosclerosis [carotid artery blockage]." As a result, he advised people "to stop taking supplemental vitamin C for any supposed cardiovascular benefit."[10]

A French study published in 2007 in *The Journal of Nutrition* found that vitamin C offered no protection against skin cancer. And, at least in women, vitamin C had the potential to increase the risk of skin cancer. Over the course of about seven and one-half years, almost 7,900 women and more than 5,100 men took 120 milligrams of vitamin C or another antioxidant or a placebo. Women in the antioxidant groups were found to have higher rates of all types of cancer, including melanoma, the most serious type of this disease.[11]

If people decide to take vitamin C, what is the recommended dosage? The federal government advises 75 milligrams for women and 90 milligrams for men. Smokers and women who are pregnant need to add more. They should check with their health care providers. In his book, *Eating Well for Optimum Health*, which was published in 2000, Andrew Weil, the director of the Program in Integrative Medicine at the University of Arizona, writes that he takes about 100 milligrams twice daily. In *Antioxidants Against Cancer*, which was also published in 2000, Ralph W. Moss says, "At a minimum, I suggest that you get at least 250 milligrams of vitamin C per day, in divided doses. 500 milligrams per day would be even better."[12]

VITAMIN E

For many years, the fat-soluble vitamin E seemed to be everyone's perfect supplement. Supporters of vitamin E found associations between it and reductions in heart disease, improved immunity, and prevention of Alzheimer's disease and cancer. Besides, people said that it may well be useful in fighting aging, Parkinson's disease, male infertility, macular degeneration, asthma, diabetes, and allergies. Some thought it might promote skin health, the healing of wounds, and it even may help deal with menopause. In *Antioxidants Against Cancer*, Ralph Moss describes a study conducted in Switzerland that found "older people who took vitamin E supplements daily were 41 percent less likely to die of cancer, and 40 percent less likely to die of heart disease, than people who did not take vitamin E."[13]

While the vast majority of studies published in the 1990s were highly supportive of vitamin E, by 1999–2000, there were a few red flags. A brief article published in early 2000 in *The Lancet* raised at least a minor caution. It described an investigation of 2,545 women and 6,996 men, aged fifty-five or older, who were at high risk for cardiovascular problems, and it found that those "who took vitamin E for a mean of 4.5 years fared no better than control in terms of cardiovascular outcome."[14]

Another study discussed in a 2000 issue of *Science News* described researchers who divided a strain of mice that developed brain tumors into two groups. One was fed a regular diet; the second was fed a diet devoid of vitamins A and E. The tumors in the mice who ate the food without vitamins A and E were half the size of the tumors in the other mice. "Moreover, 20 percent of the tumor cells in the antioxidant-deprived mice were undergoing a type of cell death called apoptosis, which is driven by free radicals. The body ordinarily uses this programmed suicide to rid itself of old or wounded cells. In the mice on the normal diet, just three percent of cancer cells were undergoing apoptosis."[15] Thus, it appeared that the antioxidants aided the growth of cancer cells.[16]

In 2000 the *New England Journal of Medicine* published a study entitled, "Vitamin E Supplementation and Cardiovascular Events in High-Risk Patients." During the study, researchers enrolled thousands of men and women fifty-five years of age or older who were at high risk for cardiovascular events. For four to six years, some people received either 400 IU of daily vitamin E from natural sources or matching placebo and either an angiotensin-converting-enzyme inhibitor (ramipril, which is used for high blood pressure) or a matching placebo. Researchers found "no significant differences in the incidence of secondary cardiovascular outcomes or in death from any cause."[17]

In an attempt to address some of the confusion concerning vitamin E, researchers at the Cleveland Clinic conducted an overview study of some of the best research on the topic. Their results were published in 2003 in *The Lancet*. In total, researchers reviewed studies on thousands of people who received doses of vitamin E ranging from 50 to 800 IU, as well as doses of beta-carotene, another antioxidant. The researchers concluded that there was a "lack of a salutary effects ... for various doses of vitamins in diverse populations." Furthermore, their "results, combined with the lack of mechanistic data for efficacy of vitamin E, do not support the routine use of vitamin E."[18] It should be parenthetically noted that beta carotene antioxidants were associated with a slight increase in mortality and cardiovascular death.

Responding to these and other published articles, in 2005, a number of researchers wrote an article entitled "Vitamin E and C Are Safe Across a Broad Range of Intakes" that appeared in the *American Journal of Clinical Nutrition*. The article notes that "because these nutrients [vitamins E and C] supply antioxidant and other functions for homeostatis and protection against free radical damage, supplementation has been intensively studied." Yet, "many clinical trials with these vitamins have involved subjects with various disease, and no consistent pattern of adverse effects has occurred at any intake." The researchers added that the Food Nutrition Board, Institute of Medicine, has indicated that adults should take no more than 1,000 milligrams of vitamin E and 2,000 milligrams of vitamin C each day.[19]

Then, in 2007 the results of a study entitled "Mortality in Randomized Trials of Supplements for Primary and Secondary Prevention" appeared in *Journal of the American Medical Association*. The research for the paper involved reviewing sixty-eight randomized trials of vitamin E and other antioxidants, including vitamin C, beta carotene, vitamin A, and selenium, with 232,606 participants—a total of 385 publications. The researchers "did not find convincing evidence that antioxidant supplements have beneficial effects on mortality. Even more, beta carotene, vitamin A, and vitamin E seem to increase the risk of death."[20]

Weeks after this study was published, in "Another Supplement, Under the Microscope," an article published in *The New York Times*, author Michael Mason noted, "for most of us, the time has come to let go of the notion that high-dose supplements provide a magic wand against disease. The good news is that a diet rich in fruits and vegetables contains literally thousands of antioxidant nutrients. Prevention begins in the kitchen."[21]

And, a few months later, in an article in *Better Nutrition*, health writer Jack Challem challenged the *Journal of the American Medical Association* article. After noting that he has been taking antioxidant supplements for thirty-eight years, Challem contended that the study was poorly designed. "On closer examination, the findings were statistically insignificant, and the researchers had no idea why people died. In fact, many of the subjects were already critically ill." But, according to Challem, there were even more problems with the study. "The researchers tried to cover too many nutrients, and dosages that were all over the map. They lumped together studies using natural and synthetic antioxidants, lasting anywhere from one day to several years. They also ignored antioxidant studies in which no deaths occurred."[22]

COENZYME Q10

Another well-publicized antioxidant is coenzyme Q10. Although its name is a bit unusual, coenzyme Q10 (also known as ubiquinone) is a naturally occurring material that is found in almost all cells of the human body. It is also contained in foods such as the following: beef hearts, liver, brain, kidney, pork, sardines, nuts, soybean oil, salmon, broccoli, spinach, and anchovies. However, some people maintain that the amount consumed from dietary sources is insufficient, especially in those dealing with illnesses such as high blood pressure and heart disease.

The literature contains numerous reports of positive outcomes facilitated by coenzyme Q10. Some of these are summarized in a 2005 article written by Robert Alan Bonakdar and Erminia Guarneri for *American Family Physician*. The authors note that much of the research on coenzyme Q10 has focused on its use for congestive heart failure (CHF). These studies have had mixed results, but there is some evidence that coenzyme Q10 may be useful for hypertension (high blood pressure) and atherosclerosis.

Bonakdar and Guarneri cite a study in which eighty people with Parkinson's disease took 1,200 milligrams per day of coenzyme Q10. They experienced "up to a 44 percent less functional decline." Another study of twenty-eight people with Parkinson's disease "demonstrated mild symptom improvement with daily oral dosing of 360 mg."[23]

In a study entitled "Atorvastatin Decreases the Coenzyme Q10 in the Blood of Patients at Risk for Cardiovascular Disease and Stroke," published in 2004 in the *Archives of Neurology*, researchers attempted to determine if coenzyme Q10 could reduce the side effects associated with the statin (cholesterol lowering) medications, such as exercise intolerance and muscle pain. Researchers at Columbia University tested the Q10 levels in thirty-four people before and after taking a daily pill containing eighty milligrams of atorvastatin. The researchers found "a highly significant and marked (about 50%) decrease in the CoQ10 concentration after two weeks of atorvastatin administration, which was essentially unchanged after four weeks of treatment." According to the researchers, "this is the first unequivocal demonstration that atorvastatin ... reduces blood levels of CoQ10...." As a result, the researchers suggested that patients placed on statin medication, especially atorvastatin, be advised to take supplemental coenzyme Q10.[24]

A study completed in the United Kingdom and Germany and published in *Circulation* in 2004 attempted to determine if coenzyme Q10 (as well as hypothermia or lowering the temperature of the body) could improve the survival rate of people who had heart attacks outside the hospital setting. Forty-nine patients were randomly assigned to have their body temperature lowered and to be treated with or without coenzyme Q10. The researchers found "a significant increase in 3-month survival after out-of-hospital cardiac arrest for patients given CoQ10 in addition to mild hypothermia, compared with patients treated with hypothermia alone." Thus, the researchers concluded that "combining CoQ10 with mild hypothermia immediately after CPR [cardio-pulmonary resuscitation] appears to improve survival and may improve neurological outcome in survivors."[25]

OTHER ANTIOXIDANTS

While vitamins C and E and coenzyme Q10 are the antioxidants that appear to generate the most publicity, there are a host of others that are discussed and, sometimes, investigated. The number of different antioxidants just keeps increasing.

Tea

One well-known and relatively inexpensive antioxidant is tea. In fact, tea is the second most consumed drink in the world. Only water is more common. Green and black teas contain polyphenols, which are powerful antioxidants that may well offer protection against high cholesterol, heart disease, and cancer. According to Marcello Spinella in *Concise Handbook of Psychoactive Herbs*, which was published in 2005, green and black tea are derived from the same plant. With green tea, the leaves are dried after they are picked; with black tea the leaves are picked and fermented before they are dried.[26] In 2003 in an article in *Original Internist*, octogenarian researcher John Weisburger summarized some of the benefits of green and black tea. Weisburger noted that population studies in Europe have found that drinkers of black tea have lower rates of heart disease. "Heart disease decreased 11% by intake of five cups (about 700 ml) of tea per day." Meanwhile, in Japan, the relative risk of cardiovascular disease and cancers were significantly lower with 10 cups of tea per day."[27] That is a huge amount of tea to drink in one day, and if it contains caffeine, it may result in restlessness, insomnia, and anxiety.

Weisburger explained that a good deal of research has found associations between tea drinking and lowered rates of cancers. For example, though Japan has more cigarette smokers than the United States, it has fewer cases of lung cancers.[28]

A study on the Dutch population published in 2002 in the *American Journal of Clinical Nutrition* found that tea drinkers were less likely to die from heart attacks. The researchers concluded, "an increased intake of tea and flavonoids may contribute to the primary prevention of ischemic heart disease [reduction in blood supply to heart]."[29] Another study published in 2007 in the same journal found an association between elderly women who drink tea and preservation of the hip structure. Researchers concluded that, "this finding provides further evidence of the beneficial effects of tea consumption on the skeleton."[30]

A Swedish study published in 2005 in the *Archives of Internal Medicine* reviewed the association between tea consumption and the risk of ovarian cancer in 61,057 women between the ages of forty and seventy-six. "During an average follow-up of 15.1 years, 301 incident cases of invasive epithelial ovarian cancer were ascertained. Tea consumption was inversely associated with the risk of ovarian cancer."[31]

There also is some potential good news for the millions of people who want to drop some weight. A study conducted in Taiwan found "habitual tea drinkers for more than 10 years showed a 19.6% reduction in BF [body fat] and a 2.1% reduction in WHR [waist-to-hip ratio] compared with nonhabitual tea drinkers."[32]

Yet, not all research on tea has had positive results. A study that appeared in 2007 in the journal *Metabolism* attempted to determine if tea could help people with type 2 diabetes achieve better control over their glucose (sugar) levels. At the end of the study, no significant difference was observed.[33]

In an investigation conducted at Beth Israel Deaconess Medical Center in Boston, Massachusetts, and published in 2007 in the *American Heart Journal*, researchers studied adults aged fifty-five years or older with diabetes or two other cardiovascular risk factors. For six months, one group drank three glasses of black tea each day; the other group drank water. The researchers found that the "black tea did not appreciably influence any traditional or novel biomarkers of cardiovascular risk."[34]

Blueberries

An American favorite, blueberries are also known to be a fruit with one of the highest levels of antioxidants. This is because blueberries contain the phytochemicals anthocyanins, phenolic acids, and other flavonoid compounds.

A 2005 article in *Nutrition Today* states that "the total antioxidant capacity of blueberries ... is twice that of spinach and three times that of oranges.... Bilberry and lowbush blueberries from Nova Scotia have the highest antioxidant capacity."[35]

There is some evidence that blueberries may help reverse aging. A study published in 2005 in *AGE* examined how blueberry, cranberry, black currant, and boysenberry supplementation affected the aging of rats. The researchers found that "antioxidants from berryfruit diets help improve neuronal functioning ... [and] restore the protective ability of the brain against oxidative or inflammatory stressor. However, the effects of each berryfruit are modulated differently, and this is presumably a result of the variety of phytochemicals in each berryfruit."[36]

In his 2004 book *The Perricone Promise*, Nicholas Perricone, a dermatologist, contends that blueberries allow the body to release the neurotransmitter dopamine, which is useful for energizing and stimulating. Blueberries also protect against the loss of dopamine cells that occurs with aging. "By increasing brain energy production and maintaining youthful brain function, dopamine exerts an extremely important anti-aging function."[37]

Ginkgo

The antioxidant ginkgo, also known as ginkgo biloba extract, kew tree, or maidenhair tree, has been featured in scientific journals and in all forms of the written and televised media. Ginkgo, which is derived from the leaves of the ginkgo tree, has ancient roots. According to the National Center for Complementary and Alternative Medicine, ginkgo has been used to treat "a variety of ailments and conditions including, asthma, bronchitis, fatigue, and tinnitus (ringing in the ears)." In addition, ginkgo has been used to improve memory, to treat or help prevent Alzheimer's disease and other types of dementia, to decrease leg pain (caused by narrowed arteries), and to treat sexual dysfunction, multiple sclerosis, tinnitus, and other health conditions.[38]

Some of the data seem to be significant. For instance, a 2000 article in *Psychology Today* noted that when daily doses of ginkgo ranging from 120 to 240 milligrams were given to thirty-one healthy people between the ages of thirty and fifty-nine, researchers observed a "slight increase in memory among those that took the ginkgo." Moreover, "the effect [was] most highly pronounced in subjects 50 to 59 years old."[39] A double-blind study of 165 women published in 2000 in *Better Nutrition* found "that ginkgo was effective in significantly reducing breast tenderness prior to menses.... The ginkgo group fared far better in terms of breast symptoms than did the placebo group."[40]

A study published in 2005 in *The Journal of Nutrition* noted that ginkgo has a number of the properties found in anticancer agents. As a result, researchers wondered if it may be effective against prostate cancer. In laboratory experimentation, it was found to inhibit the growth of prostate cancer cells. Researchers concluded that "ginkgo may be a chemopreventive as well as chemotherapeutic agent for prostate cancer management and provide rationale to further test this innovative idea in animal models and clinical studies."[41]

On the other hand, an article published in 2002 in *Journal of the American Medical Association* describes a six-week, randomized, double-blind, placebo-controlled study in which ginkgo was tested in more than 200 men and women over the age of sixty. Researchers found that "ginkgo provides no measurable benefit in memory or relative cognitive function to adults with healthy cognitive function."[42]

Of even more concern is a report, published in 2006 in *Healthy Years,* indicating that a number of brands of ginkgo have been found to contain significant amounts of lead. A business known as consumerlab.com tested thirteen brands of ginkgo. "Only six products ... had ingredients that passed standards for purity, quantity, and proper identification."[43]

Different people recommend varying amounts of ginkgo. Most studies tend to advise 120 milligrams per day, divided into two or three doses. However, a warning needs to be noted. People who are taking blood-thinning medications, such as warfarin or high-dose aspirin, should avoid ginkgo; otherwise, they are at risk for developing bleeding problems. Other possible side effects of ginkgo include nausea, diarrhea, leg pain, dizziness, headaches, gastrointestinal problems, and/ or allergic skin reactions. On occasion, there have been severe allergic reactions. Unprocessed ginkgo leaves, which contain allergens, should never be used. During processing, the allergens are removed.

Acai

Although the acai berry (*Euterpe oleraceae*) has been a staple of the Brazilian diet for centuries, over the past few years this Amazonian antioxidant has been generating quite a bit of attention. Why? Because the acai berry (pronounced ah-sigh-EE) has extraordinarily high levels of antioxidants and cholesterol-fighting fatty acids. It is now considered a "superfood." A 2007 article in *Chemistry and Industry* outlined some of the positive aspects of acai. "Acai is a rich source of a class of polyphenolic flavonoids called anthocyanins—the same antioxidants that give wine its health benefits. As well as being a good source of antioxidants, acai is rich in mono-and polyunsaturated fatty acids including omega 6 and 9. It also contains phytosterols, which can help the body prevent the absorption of cholesterol."[44]

A study completed at the University of Florida and published in 2006 in the *Journal of Agricultural and Food Chemistry* found that extracts of acai caused a self-destruct response in up to 86 percent of the leukemia cells that were tested. While this research may ultimately prove to be significant, it is important to note that the researchers worked with a cell-culture model.[45]

Chocolate

While many high-antioxidant foods are fruits and vegetables, one surprising antioxidant is chocolate. According to a 2007 article in *Critical Care Nurse,* "chocolate is derived from the cocoa bean, one of the most concentrated sources of flavanols, a subgroup of the natural antioxidant plants compounds called flavonoids."[46] In fact, "chocolate is the third highest daily source of antioxidants for U.S. consumers."

Research has found that chocolate may well lower blood pressure, enhance blood flow, improve cognitive functioning, and reduce overall mortality. However, it is important to note that not all chocolate is equally healthful. "The health benefits ascribed to chocolate relate nearly exclusively to the dark, bittersweet tasting chocolate and to products with a cocoa content of 60% or more. As a general rule, the darker the chocolate, the more likely it is to offer health benefits."[47]

But, chocolate also contains caffeine. In fact, milk chocolate may have as much as fifteen milligrams of caffeine per ounce, and dark chocolate may have as much as thirty-five mg per ounce. According to Marcello Spinella in *Concise Handbook of Psychoactive Herbs*, "three ounces of dark chocolate has the caffeine equivalent of an average cup of coffee."[48]

CONCLUSION

It is a little unsettling to close this chapter with so many unexplained findings. Why does one study find this or that antioxidant useful when another concludes that it may be detrimental to one's health? Some have speculated that antioxidants may require certain other antioxidants and nutrients to work effectively. When these other antioxidants and nutrients are absent, the antioxidants may fail to function at optimum capacity. The overall nutritional state of the individual may also be a factor in their effectiveness.

It is of interest that in a 2006 article in *New Scientist,* science writer, Lisa Melton, advises people not to take antioxidant supplements. "Not only are they bad at preventing oxidative damage, they can even make things worse. Many scientists are now concluding that, at best, they are a waste of time and money. At worse, they could be harmful. . . . Whatever is behind the health benefits of a diet rich in fruits and vegetables, you cannot reproduce it by taking purified extracts or vitamin supplements."[49]

While the issues surrounding antioxidants remain controversial, it is obvious that many people could increase their intake simply by adding more fruits and vegetables to their daily diet and maybe, even, a small piece of dark chocolate. For most people, those are probably the easiest and most effective lifestyle modifications.

TOPICS FOR DISCUSSION

1. Before reading this chapter, did you know what antioxidants were? Summarize what you have learned about them in one paragraph.
2. Have you ever taken high doses of vitamin C to prevent a cold? What happened? Did you still develop the cold? Was it milder than most of your colds? Do you believe that high doses of vitamin C are useful? Why or why not?

3. Do you think that antioxidant supplements may be harmful? Why or why not?

4. After reading this chapter, do you think you will take any antioxidant supplements? Why or why not?

5. After reading this chapter, did you make any modifications in your diet? If you did, please describe the changes.

NOTES

1. Estitta Bushkin and Gary Bushkin, "Anti-Aging with Antioxidants," *Better Nutrition* (February 2000) 6: 66–70.

2. U.S. Department of Agriculture website, http://www.usda.gov.

3. Jean Carper, *Your Miracle Brain* (New York: HarperCollins Publishers, 2000), 249.

4. Ping Gao, Huafeng Zhang, Ramani Dinavahi, Feng Li, Yan Xiang, Venu Raman, Zaver M. Bhuywalla, Dean W. Felsher, Linzhao Cheng, Jonathan Pevsner, Linda A. Lee, Gregg L. Semenza, and Chi V. Dang, "HIF-Dependent Antitumorigenic Effect of Antioxidants in Vivo," *Cancer Cell* (September 11, 2007) 12: 230–8.

5. "Reducing Stress with Vitamin C," *USA Today* (Magazine) (October 2002) 131: 10.

6. Masao Yoshida, Yutaka Takashima, Manami Inoue, Motoki Iwasaki, Tetsuya Otani, Satoshi Sasaki, and Shoichiro Tsugane, "Prospective Study Showing that Dietary Vitamin C Reduced the Risk of Age-Related Cataracts in A Middle-Aged Japanese Population," *European Journal of Nutrition* (March 2007) 46: 118–24.

7. Gladys Block, Christopher Jensen, Marion Dietrich, Edward P. Norkus, Mark Hudes, and Lester Packer, "Plasma C-Reactive Protein Concentrations in Active and Passive Smokers: Influence of Antioxidant Supplementation," *Journal of the American College of Nutrition* (April 2004) 23: 141–7.

8. Nancy R. Cook, Christine M. Albert, J. Michael Gaziano, Elaine Zaharris, Jean MacFadyen, Eleanor Danielson, Julie E. Buring, and JoAnn E. Manson, "A Randomized Factorial Trial of Vitamin C and E and Beta Carotene in the Secondary Prevention of Cardiovascular Events," *Archives of Internal Medicine* (August 13/27, 2007) 167: 1610–18.

9. Ian D. Coulter, Mary L. Hardy, Sally C. Morton, Lara G. Hilton, Wenli Tu, Di Valentine, and Paul G. Shekelle, "Antioxidants Vitamin C and E for the Prevention and Treatment of Cancer," *Journal of General Internal Medicine* (July 2006) 21: 735–44.

10. Bruce Jancin, "Vitamin C Supplements May Accelerate Atherosclerosis," *Family Practice News* (May 15, 2000) 30: 17.

11. Serge Hercberg, Khaled Ezzedine, Christine Guinot, Paul Preziosi, Pilar Galan, Sandrine Bertrais, Carla Estaquio, Serge Briancon, Alain Favier, Julie Latreille, and Denis Malvy, "Antioxidant Supplementation Increases the Risk of Skin Cancers in Women But Not In Men," *The Journal of Nutrition* (September 2007) 137: 2098–105.

12. Ralph W. Moss, *Antioxidants Against Cancer* (Brooklyn, New York: Equinox Press, 2000) 50.

13. Moss, *Anitoxidants Against Cancer*, 53.

14. Kathryn Senior, "Setback for Vitamin E as Preventive Therapy for Cardiovascular Disease," *The Lancet* (January 29, 2000) 355: 383.

15. Janet Raloff, "Antioxidants May Help Cancers Thrive," *Science News* (January 1, 2000) 157: 11.

16. Rudolf I. Salganik, Craig D. Albright, Jerilyn Rodgers, John Kim, Steven H. Zeisel, Mikhail S. Sivashinskiy, and Terry A. Van Dyke, "Dietary Antioxidant Depletion: Enhancement of Tumor Apoptosis and Inhibition of Brain Tumor Growth in Transgenic Mice," *Carcinogenesis* (May 2000) 21: 909–14.

17. Salim Yusaf, Gilles Dagenais, Janice Pogue, Jackie Bosch, and Peter Sleight, "Vitamin E Supplementation and Cardiovascular Events in High-Risk Patients," *New England Journal of Medicine* (January 20, 2000) 342: 154–60.

18. Deepak Vivekananthan, Marc S. Penn, Shelly K. Sapp, Amy Hsu, and Eric J. Topol, "Use of Antioxidant Vitamins for the Prevention of Cardiovascular Disease: Meta-Analysis of Randomised Trials," *The Lancet* (June 14, 2003) 361: 2017–23.

19. John N. Hathcock, Angelo Azzi, Jeffrey Blumberg, Tammy Bray, Annette Dickinson, Balz Frei, Ishwarial Jialal, Carol S. Johnston, Frank J. Kelly, Klaus Kraemer, Lester Packer, Sampath Parthasarathy, Helmut Sies, and Maret G. Traber, "Vitamin E and C Are Safe Across a Broad Range of Intakes," *Journal of Clinical Nutrition* (April 2005) 81(4): 736–45.

20. Goran Bjelakovic, Dimitrinka Nikolova, Lise Lotte Gluud, Rosa G. Simonetti, and Christian Gluud, "Mortality in Randomized Trials of Antioxidant Supplements for Primary and Secondary Prevention," *Journal of the American Medical Association* (February 28, 2007) 297: 842–57.

21. Michael Mason, "Another Supplement, Under the Microscope," *The New York Times* (March 13, 2007) F5.

22. Jack Challem, "Are Antioxidants Still Safe? Were Important Details Omitted from a Recent Study on Antioxidants? A Closer Look Reveals the Real Story," *Better Nutrition* (May 2007) 69: 16.

23. Robert Alan Bonakdar and Erminia Guarneri, "Coenzyme Q10," *American Family Physician* (September 15, 2005) 72: 1065–70.

24. Tatjana Rundek, Ali Naini, Ralph Sacco, Kristen Coates, and Salvatore DiMaura, "Atorvastatin Decreases the Coenzyme Q10 Levels in the Blood of Patients at Risk for Cardiovascular Disease and Stroke," *Archives of Neurology* (June 2004) 61: 889–92.

25. Maxwell Simon Damian, Diana Ellenberg, Ramona Gildemeister, Jörg Lauermann, Gregor Simonis, Wolfgang Sauter, and Christian Georgi, "Coenzyme Q10 Combined with Mild Hypothermia After Cardiac Arrest: A Preliminary Study," *Circulation* (November 9, 2004) 110: 3011–6.

26. Marcello Spinella, *Concise Handbook of Psychoactive Herbs* (Binghamton, New York: The Haworth Press) 42.

27. John H. Weisburger, "Regular Intake of Tea Can Decrease the Risk of Heart Disease and Several Types of Cancer and Provides Basis for Improved Aging," *Original Internist* (September 2003) 10: 25–8.

28. Weisburger, "Regular Intake of Tea."

29. Johanna M. Geleijnse, Lenore J. Launer, Deirdre AM. van der Kuip, Albert Hoffman, and Jacqueline CM. Witteman, "Inverse Association of Tea

and Flavonoid Intakes with Incident Myocardial Infarction: the Rotterdam Study," *American Journal of Clinical Nutrition* (May 2002) 75: 880–6.

30. Amanda Devine, Jonathan M. Hodgson, Ian M. Dick, and Richard L. Price, "Tea Drinking is Associated with Benefits on Bone Density in Older Women," *American Journal of Clinical Nutrition* (October 2007) 86: 1243–7.

31. Susanna C. Larsson and Alicja Wolk, "Tea Consumption and Ovarian Cancer Risk in a Population-Based Cohort," *Archives of Internal Medicine* (December 12/26, 2005) 165: 2683–6.

32. Chih-Hsing Wu, Feng-Hwa Lu, Chin-Song Chang, Tsui-Chen Chang, Ru-Hsueh Wang, and Chih-Jen Chang, "Relationship Among Habitual Tea Consumption, Percent Body Fat, and Body Fat Distribution," *Obesity* (September 2003) 11: 1088–95.

33. Todd MacKenzie, Lisa Leary, and W. Blair Brooks, "The Effect of An Extract of Green and Black Tea on Glucose Control in Adults with Type 2 Diabetes Mellitus: Double-Blind Randomized Study," *Metabolism* (October 2007) 56: 1340–4.

34. Kenneth J. Mukamal, Kristen MacDermott, Joe A. Vinson, Noriko Oyama, Warren J. Manning, and Murray A. Mittleman, "A 6-Month Randomized Pilot Study of Black Tea and Cardiovascular Risk Factors," *American Heart Journal* (October 2007) 154: 724.e1–724.e6.

35. Nancy M. Lewis and Jaime Ruud, "Blueberries in the American Diet," *Nutrition Today* (March-April 2005) 40: 92–6.

36. Barbara Shukitt-Hale, Rachel L. Galli, Vanessa Meterko, Amanda Carey, Donna F. Bielinski, Tony McGhie, and James A. Joseph, "Dietary Supplementation with Fruit Polyphenolics Ameliorates Age-Related Deficits in Behavior and Neuronal Markers of Inflammation and Oxidative Stress," *AGE* (March 2005) 27: 49–57.

37. Nicholas Perricone, *The Perricone Promise* (New York: Warner Books), 55.

38. National Center for Complementary and Alternative Medicine, website: http://nccam.nih.gov

39. "Ginkgo: The End of Alzheimer's Disease?" *Psychology Today* (March 2000) 33: 46.

40. J. Jamison Starbuck, "Beyond Brainboosting," *Better Nutrition* (April 2000) 62: 72.

41. Wen Wang, Luzhe Sun, Ian Thompson, and Linda deGraffenried, "A Novel Strategy Using Ginkgo Biloba Extract for the Chemoprevention of Prostate Cancer," *The Journal of Nutrition* (December 2005) 135: 3049S.

42. Paul R. Solomon, Felicity Adams, Amanda Silver, Jill Zimmer, and Richard DeVeaux. "Ginkgo for Memory Enhancement," *Journal of the American Medical Association* (August 21, 2002) 288: 835–40.

43. "Your Ginkgo May Be Loaded with Lead" *Healthy Years* (March 2006) 3: 2.

44. Anna Jagger, "Amazonian Berry: On a Scale of the World's Most Nutritious and Health 'Superfoods,' the Brazilian Acai Berry is Claimed to Rank Alongside Blueberries, and Pomegranates for its Health-Giving Properties," *Chemistry and Industry* (March 26, 2007) 6: 24–5.

45. David del Pozo-Insfran, Susan S. Percival, and Stephen T. Talcott. "Acai (*Euterpe oleracea* Mart.) Polyphenolics in Their Glycoside and Aglycone Forms

Induce Apoptosis of HL-60 Leukemia Cells," *Journal of Agriculture and Food Chemistry* (January 12, 2006) 54(4): 1222–9.

46. Grif Alspach, "The Truth Is Often Bittersweet ... Chocolate Does a Heart Good," *Critical Care Nurse* (February 2007) 27: 11–14.

47. Alspach, "The Truth Is Often Bittersweet."

48. Marcello Spinella, *Concise Handbook of Psychoactive Herbs* (Binghamton, New York: The Haworth Press, 2005), 44.

49. Lisa Melton, "The Antioxidant Myth: If Popping Pills to Stave Off the Ravages of Aging Sounds Too Good to Be True, That's Because It Is," *New Scientist* (August 5, 2006) 191: 40–43.

REFERENCES AND RESOURCES

Books

Carper, Jean. *Your Miracle Brain.* New York: HarperCollins Publishers, 2000.

Keane, Maureen and Danielle Chace. *What to Eat If You Have Cancer.* New York: McGraw Hill, 2007.

Meletis, Chris Demetrios and Jason E. Barker. *Herbs and Nutrients for the Mind.* Westport, Connecticut: Praeger, 2004.

Moss, Ralph. *Antioxidants Against Cancer.* Brooklyn, New York: Equinox Press, 2000.

Perricone, Nicholas. *The Perricone Promise.* New York: Warner Books, 2004.

Spinella, Marcello. *Concise Handbook of Psychoactive Herbs.* Binghamton, New York: The Haworth Press, 2005.

Weil, Andrew. *Eating Well for Optimum Health.* New York: Alfred Knopf, 2000.

Magazines, Journals, and Newspapers

Alspach, Grif. "The Truth Is Often Bittersweet ... Chocolate Does a Heart Good." *Critical Care Nurse* (February 2007) 27: 11–14.

Andersen-Parrado, Patricia. "Vitamin C: Friend or Foe?" *Better Nutrition* (June 2000): NA.

Bjelakovic, Goran, Dimitrinka Nikolova, Lise Lotte Gluud, Rosa G. Simonetti, and Christian Gluud. "Mortality in Randomized Trials of Antioxidant Supplements for Primary and Secondary Prevention." *Journal of the American Medical Association* (February 28, 2007) 297: 842–56.

Block, Gladys, Christopher Jensen, Marion Dietrich, Edward P. Norkus, Mark Hudes, and Lester Packer. "Plasma C-Reactive Protein Concentrations in Active and Passive Smokers: Influence of Antioxidant Supplementation." *Journal of the American College of Nutrition* (April 2004) 23: 141–7.

Bonakdar, Robert Alan and Erminia Guarneri. "Coenzyme Q10." *American Family Physician* (September 15, 2005) 72: 1065–70.

Bushkin, Estitta and Gary Bushkin. "Anti-Aging with Antioxidants." *Better Nutrition* (February 2000) 6: 66–70.

Challem, Jack. "Are Antioxidants Still Safe? Were Important Details Omitted from a Recent Study on Antioxidants? A Closer Look Reveals the Real Story." *Better Nutrition* (May 2007) 69: 16.

Cook, Nancy R., Christine M. Albert, J. Michael Gaziano, Elaine Zaharris, Jean MacFadyen, Eleanor Danielson, Julie E. Buring, and JoAnn E. Manson. "A Randomized Factorial Trial of Vitamins C and E and Beta Carotene in the Secondary Prevention of Cardiovascular Events." *Archives of Internal Medicine* (August 13/27, 2007) 167: 1610–18.

Coulter, Ian D., Mary L. Hardy, Sally C. Morton, Lara G. Hilton, Wenli Tu, Di Valentine, and Paul G. Shekelle. "Antioxidants Vitamin C and E for the Prevention and Treatment of Cancer." *Journal of General Internal Medicine* (July 2006) 21: 735–44.

Damian, Maxwell Simon, Diana Ellenberg, Ramona Gildemeister, Jörg Lauermann, Gregor Simonis, Wolfgang Sauter, and Christian Georgi. "Coenzyme Q10 Combined with Mild Hypothermia after Cardiac Arrest: A Preliminary Study." *Circulation* (November 9, 2004) 110: 3011–16.

del Pozo-Insfran, David, Susan S. Percival, and Stephen T. Talcott. "Acai (*Euterpe oleracea* Mart.) Polyphenolics in Their Glycoside and Aglycone Forms Induce Apoptosis of HL-60 Leukemia Cells." *Journal of Agricultural and Food Chemistry* (January 12, 2006) 54: 1222–9.

Devine, Amanda, Jonathan M. Hodgson, Ian M. Dick, and Richard L. Prince. "Tea Drinking Is Associated with Benefits on Bone Density in Older Women." *American Journal of Clinical Nutrition* (October 2007) 86: 1243–7.

Gao, Ping, Huafeng Zhang, Ramani Dinavahi, Feng Li, Yan Xiang, Venu Raman, Zaver M. Bhuywalla, Dean W. Felsher, Linzhao Cheng, Jonathan Pevsner, Linda A. Lee, Gregg L. Semenza, and Chi V. Dang. "HIF-Dependent Antitumorigenic Effect of Antioxidants in Vivo." *Cancer Cell* (September 11, 2007) 12: 230–8.

Geleijnse, Johanna M., Lenore J. Launer, Deirdre AM. van der Kuip, Albert Hoffman, and Jacqueline CM. Witteman. "Inverse Association of Tea and Flavonoid Intakes with Incident Myocardial Infarction: The Rotterdam Study." *American Journal of Clinical Nutrition* (May 2002) 75: 880–6.

"Ginkgo: The End of Alzheimer's Disease?" *Psychology Today* (March 2000) 33: 46.

Hathcock, John N., Angelo Azzi, Jeffrey Blumberg, Tammy Bray, Annette Dickinson, Balz Frei, Ishwarial Jialal, Carol S. Johnston, Frank J. Kelly, Klaus Kraemer, Lester Packer, Sampath Parthasarathy, Helmut Sies, and Maret G. Traber. "Vitamins E and C Are Safe Across a Broad Range of Intakes." *Journal of Clinical Nutrition* (April 2005) 81: 736–45.

Hercberg, Serge, Khaled Ezzedine, Christiane Guinot, Paul Preziosi, Pilar Galan, Sandrine Bertrais, Carla Estaquio, Serge Briancon, Alain Favier, Julie Latreille, and Denis Malvy. "Antioxidant Supplementation Increases the Risk of Skin Cancers in Women But Not In Men." *The Journal of Nutrition* (September 2007) 137: 2098–105.

Jagger, Anna. "Amazonian Berry: On a Scale of the World's Most Nutritious and Health 'Superfoods,' the Brazilian Acai Berry Is Claimed to Rank Alongside Blueberries, and Pomegranates for its Health-Giving Properties." *Chemistry and Industry* (March 26, 2007) 6: 24–5.

Jancin, Bruce. "Vitamin C Supplements May Accelerate Atherosclerosis." *Family Practice News* (May 15, 2000) 30: 17.

Larsson, Susanna C. and Alicja Wolk. "Tea Consumption and Ovarian Cancer Risk in a Population-Based Cohort." *Archives of Internal Medicine* (December 12/26, 2005) 165: 2683–6.

Lewis, Nancy M. and Jaime Ruud. "Blueberries in the American Diet." *Nutrition Today* (March-April 2005) 40: 92–6.

MacKenzie, Todd, Lisa Leary, and W. Blair Brooks. "The Effect of An Extract of Green and Black Tea on Glucose Control in Adults with Type 2 Diabetes Mellitus: Double-Blind Randomized Study." *Metabolism* (October 2007) 56: 1340–4.

Mason, Michael. "Another Supplement, Under the Microscope." *The New York Times* (March 13, 2007): F5.

Melton, Lisa. "The Antioxidant Myth: If Popping Pills to Stave Off the Ravages of Aging Sounds Too Good to Be True, That's Because It Is." *New Scientist* (August 5, 2006) 191: 40–3.

Mukamal, Kenneth J., Kristen MacDermott, Joe A. Vinson, Noriko Oyama, Warren J. Manning, and Murray A. Mittleman. "A 6-Month Randomized Pilot Study of Black Tea and Cardiovascular Risk Factors." *American Heart Journal* (October 2007) 154: 724.e1–724.e6.

Raloff, Janet. "Antioxidants May Help Cancers Thrive." *Science News* (January 1, 2000) 157: 11.

"Reducing Stress with Vitamin C." *USA Today* (Magazine) (October 2002) 131: 10.

Ross, Stephanie Maxine. "Coenzyme Q10: Ubiquinone: A Potent Antioxidant and Key Energy Facilitator for the Heart." *Holistic Nursing Practice* (July-August 2007) 21: 213–14.

Rundek, Tatjana. Ali Naini, Ralph Sacco, Kristen Coates, and Salvatore DiMaura. "Atorvastatin Decreases the Coenzyme Q10 Level in the Blood of Patients at Risk for Cardiovascular Disease and Stroke." *Archives of Neurology* (June 2004) 61: 889–92.

Salganik, Rudolf I., Craig D. Albright, Jerilyn Rodgers, John Kim, Steven H. Zeisel, Mikhail S. Sivashinskiy, and Terry A. Van Dyke. "Dietary Antioxidant Depletion: Enhancement of Tumor Apoptosis and Inhibition of Brain Tumor Growth in Transgenic Mice." *Carcinogensis* (May 2000) 21: 909–14.

Senior, Kathryn. "Setback for Vitamin E as Preventive Therapy for Cardiovascular Disease," *The Lancet* (January 29, 2000) 355: 383.

Shukitt-Hale, Barbara, Rachel L. Galli, Vanessa Meterko, Amanda Carey, Donna F. Bielinski, Tony McGhie, and James A. Joseph. "Dietary Supplementation with Fruit Polyphenolics Ameliorates Age-Related Deficits in Behavior and Neuronal Markers of Inflammation and Oxidative Stress. *AGE* (March 2005) 27: 49–57.

Solomon, Paul R., Felicity Adams, Amanda Silver, Jill Zimmer, and Richard DeVeaux. "Ginkgo for Memory Enhancement." *Journal of the American Medical Association* (August 21, 2002) 288: 835–40.

Starbuck, J. Jamison. "Beyond Brainboosting." *Better Nutrition* (April 2000) 62: 72.

Vivekananthan, Deepak, Marc S. Penn, Shelly K. Sapp, Amy Hsu, and Eric J. Topol."Use of Antioxidant Vitamins for the Prevention of Cardiovascular Disease: Meta-Analysis of Randomised Trials." *The Lancet* (June 14, 2003) 361(9374): 2017–23.

Wang, Wen, Luzhe Sun, Ian Thompson, and Linda deGraffenried. "A Novel Strategy Using Ginkgo Biloba Extract for the Chemoprevention of Prostate Cancer." *The Journal of Nutrition* (December 2005) 135: 3049S.

Weisburger, John H. "Regular Intake of Tea Can Decrease the Risk of Heart Disease and Several Types of Cancer and Provides Basis for Improved Aging." *Original Internist* (September 2003) 10: 25–8.

Wu, Chih-Hsing, Feng-Hwa Lu, Chin-Song Chang, Tsui-Chen Chang, Ru-Hsueh Wang, and Chih-Jen Chang. "Relationship Among Habitual Tea Consumption, Percent Body Fat, and Body Fat Distribution." *Obesity* (September 2003) 11: 1088–95.

"Your Ginkgo May Be Loaded with Lead." *Healthy Years* (March 2006) 3: 2.

Yoshida, Masao, Yutaka Takashima, Manami Inoue, Motoki Iwasaki, Tetsuya Otani, Satoshi Sasaki, and Shoichiro Tsugane. "Prospective Study Showing That Dietary Vitamin C Reduced the Risk of Age-Related Cataracts in a Middle-Aged Japanese Population." *European Journal of Nutrition* (March 2007) 46: 118–24.

Yusaf, Salim, Gilles Dagenais, Janice Pogue, Jackie Bosch, and Peter Sleight. "Vitamin E Supplementation and Cardiovascular Events in High-Risk Patients." *New England Journal of Medicine* (January 20, 2000) 342: 154–60.

Websites

National Center for Complementary and Alternative Medicine
National Institutes of Health
http://nccam.nih.gov

Office of Dietary Supplements
National Institutes of Health
http://ods.od.nih.gov

U.S. Department of Agriculture
http://www.usda.gov

Chapter 2

Bottled Water or Tap?

It is often said that people should drink at least eight 8-ounce glasses of water each day. What is not so clear is whether those 64 ounces of water should be obtained by purchasing bottled water or simply opening the kitchen faucet. If you live in New York City and drink the tap water, the annual bill for your daily water will be about 49 cents. On the other hand, if you drink bottled water, you will pay a 2,900-fold premium or about $1,400 each year.[1]

Is bottled water worth the extra cost? Is it a significant improvement over tap water? And how about all those bottles? Only a small fraction of them are recycled. What is their impact on the environment? These issues have become quite controversial.

What no one denies is that bottled water is a massive industry—one that has been experiencing significant growth. According to the International Bottled Water Association, in 2006, the consumption of bottled water in the United States surpassed 8.25 billion gallons, a 9.5 percent increase over 2005. The average person drank 27.6 gallons, up more than 2 gallons from 2005. That means U.S. residents now drink more bottled water annually than any other beverage except soft drinks.[2] And the cost is extraordinary. In 2006 Americans spent nearly $11 billion on bottled water.[3] A Gallup Poll, commissioned by the Environmental Protection Agency (EPA) and conducted in 2007, found that, in the United States, one in five people drinks only bottled water.[4] As Francis H. Chapelle wrote in *Wellsprings: A Natural History of Bottle Spring Waters,* which was published in 2005, "Like the phoenix rising from the ashes, the bottled water industry has risen from obscurity to unprecedented heights of profitability."[5]

In the book *Bottlemania,* which was published in 2008, Elizabeth Royte writes that bottles of water are everywhere. "They are ubiquitous in vending machines, at newsstands, and in gas stations. Our cars, StairMasters,

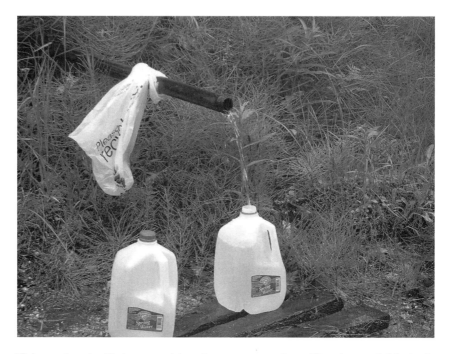

This spring in Maine provides free, pure water. (Courtesy of Mark A. Goldstein)

and movie-theater seats have been redesigned to accommodate them. Altogether, more than seven hundred domestic and seventy-five imported brands are sold in the United States."[6]

Commenting on the bottled water industry in 2007, Richard Wilk, a professor of anthropology at Indiana University, said, "This is an industry that takes free liquid that falls from the sky and sells it for as much as four times what we pay for gas. There's almost nowhere in America where the drinking water isn't adequate. Municipalities spend billions of dollars bringing clean, cheap water to people's homes. But many of us would still rather buy it at a store."[7]

At the same time, the Container Recycling Institute notes that the vast majority of the bottled water sold in the U.S. is packaged in polyethylene terephthalate (PET) plastic bottles, usually in "single serving" sizes. (PET bottles have the number 1 on the bottom.) And, most of these bottles, which are made from petroleum (oil), are not recycled. Instead, bottles are placed in the trash or left on the side of the road or thrown wherever. "In 2005, 23.1% of the 5 billion pounds of PET sold in the U.S. were recycled." This figure includes carbonated soft drinks, which are recycled more often than bottled water.[8] As a result, an overwhelming number of bottles are filling landfills. According to the

Worldwatch Institute, "each year about two million tons of PET bottles end up in landfills in the United States."[9]

Because so few bottles are recycled, the Container Recycling Institute notes that new bottles, from "virgin materials rather than bottle resin," must be made, thereby producing more greenhouse gases, a key element in global warming. "An estimated 800 thousand metric tons of carbon equivalent (MTCE) were released in the process of making approximately 50 billion new PET bottles from virgin rather than recycled materials."[10]

The toll on the environment should not be minimized. A 2007 article in *Time* magazine noted that in addition to needing oil to make plastic, oil is used to transport the bottled water from the source to the consumer, which may take thousands of miles. That also results in greenhouse gases. "The NRDC estimates that 4,000 tons of CO_2 is generated each year—the equivalent of the emissions of 700 cars—by importing bottled water from Fiji, France and Italy, three of the biggest suppliers to the U.S."[11]

Even the PET bottles themselves have garnered controversy. Many believe that they contain bisphenol A, a chemical that may disturb the body's endocrine system. But, according to the National Association for PET Container Resources (NAPCOR), a trade organization for the PET plastic industry, PET bottles do not contain bisphenol, which is actually found in sturdier plastic bottles, such as those used by bikers, hikers, and babies. NAPCOR maintains that PET bottles may be frozen or left in hot cars. Freezing and exposure to heat does not result in the leaching of chemicals. And PET bottles do not have the chemicals known as phthalates. NAPCOR does acknowledge that PET bottles contain tiny amounts of antimony, a potentially toxic trace element. It is used as a catalyst in the production of PET plastic. NAPCOR says, "Its very low toxicity combined with very low extraction rate from PET translates to very, very low risk. Its use in PET does not endanger workers, consumers, or the environment."[12]

Professor William Shotyk, of the Institute of Environmental Geochemistry at the University of Heidelberg, is not so sure that NAPCOR is correct. In two separate studies, he found that, over time, antimony may leach from PET bottles. "The amount of antimony in natural water that is not contaminated is extremely low," he has said. "The amount of antimony in bottled waters is hundreds, sometimes thousands, of times higher."[13]

Given the exorbitant expense and the toll that it exacts from the environment, it might be safe to assume that bottled water must be healthier than tap water—just as the bottled water companies want people to believe. "Not necessarily," notes the Natural Resources Defense Council (NRDC), an environmental group. After conducting a four-year study of the bottled water industry and the safety standards by which it is governed, which included the testing of more than 1,000 bottles of 103 brands of bottled water, the NRDC concluded that bottled water may not be cleaner or safer than water from the faucet. Moreover, the organization determined that about 25 percent of bottled water is actually "tap water in a bottle—sometimes further treated, sometimes not." If the bottle label or the cap says that the water is "from a municipal source" or "from a community water system," then the water was obtained from tap water.[14]

A 2007 article in *The Economist (US)* noted that PepsiCo, the maker of the bottled water Aquafina, had agreed to change the labeling on their bottles from the "innocent-looking 'P.W.S.' to the more revealing 'public water source.'" The article also noted that Coca-Cola refused to alter the labeling on Dasani, its bottled water. A spokeswoman from Coca-Cola is quoted to have said, "The label clearly states that it is purified water."[15]

During their research, the NRDC determined that about 22 percent of the brands tested contained chemical contaminants, such as synthetic organic chemicals and bacteria, above state health limits. This has potential to cause the most harm to those dealing with chronic illness, as well as infants and frail elderly.[16] Yet, these contaminants usually cannot be seen, smelled, or tasted.

One cannot help but wonder why the water produced by the bottled water industry is not more rigorously scrutinized. That is why it is important to realize that different agencies set the standards for tap and bottled water. The standards for tap water are set by the Environmental Protection Agency (EPA); the standards for bottled water, which is considered a food product, are set by the Food and Drug Administration (FDA). The EPA standards for tap water are far more rigorous than those of the FDA for bottled water. For example, the NRDC notes that bottled water is tested far less often than city tap water for bacteria and contaminants. And, though city tap water must be filtered to remove pathogens or have a strictly protected source that is not the case for bottled water. City water is required to be checked for certain toxic or cancer-causing chemicals, such as phthalate, a chemical that may leach from plastic bottles. Bottled water does not have this requisite. And, city water must be tested by government-certified laboratories. There is no such requirement for bottled water.[17]

In addition, the FDA allows the bottled water companies to practice misleading marketing. "For example," says the NRDC, "one brand of 'spring water' whose label pictured a lake and mountains, actually came from a well in an industrial facility's parking lot, near a hazardous waste dump, and periodically was contaminated with industrial chemicals at levels above FDA standards."[18] A 2007 article in *American City & County* describes how the labeling of Aquafina has snow-capped peaks, which seems to indicate that the water comes from cold mountain streams. Instead, as has been noted, it is tap water. So what do the mountains represent? Simply, "a place where PepsiCo executives can afford to vacation, such as the Alps."[19]

Furthermore, the FDA exempts some bottled water from its standards. Thus, water that is packaged and sold within the same state is exempt, as is carbonated water and seltzer. As a result, the NRDC has determined that between 60 and 70 percent of the bottled water that is sold in the United States does not need to comply with FDA standards.[20]

So how can people know what is in the bottled water they are drinking? The Environmental Working Group (EWG) cites a few labeling rules. A product described as "drinking water" must be bottled in sanitary conditions and must not contain any sweeteners or chemical additives. But it may contain flavoring. "Mineral water" has at least 250 parts per million of total dissolved naturally occurring solids. "Purified water" is usually tap water that has been filtered. And "spring water" has been obtained from a spring.[21]

Yet tap water may also have problems. In fact, it is because tap water is so frequently evaluated that problems are likely to be detected. In 2005, the EWG tested city water in 42 states and found about 260 contaminants—"140 of which were unregulated chemicals, that is, chemicals for which public health officials have no safety standards for, much less methods for removing them."[22] Fortunately, the vast majority of these are in small concentrations too small to harm the average relatively healthy person.

Then, in 2007, the EWG collected tap water samples from eighteen Washington, D.C., locations. Again, the findings were problematic. Over 40 percent of the samples had chemical water treatment by-products that exceeded federal limits. Commenting on the situation, the EWP noted, "Chlorination of tap water is one of the greatest public health improvements of the last 100 years, vastly reducing deaths from water-borne diseases. But, chlorination produces disinfection by-products (DBPs) like THMs and HAAs that are themselves potentially harmful."[23]

Still, despite the problems, cities and towns throughout the country generally provide clean and safe water for their citizens 365 days per year. Of course, some places do this better than others. According to the American Water Works Association, some of the best tasting water in the country may be found in St. Louis, Missouri, Annheim, California, Colorado Springs, Colorado, Long Beach, California, and Toledo, Ohio.

A number of U.S. mayors are beginning to ask for limitations in the use of bottled water. In 2006 Rocky Anderson, the mayor of Salt Lake City, requested that city officials discontinue the practice of handing out bottled water at meetings and events. Then, in 2007 Gavin Newscom, the mayor of San Francisco, signed a bill that banned city offices from purchasing bottled water, "mandating instead that city departments rely on tap water that gushes down to the city from its clean reservoirs in Yosemite National Park."[24] Newscom noted that "more than one billion plastic water bottles end up in California's landfills every year, taking 1000 years to biodegrade and leaking toxic additives such as phthalates into the ground water."[25] Around the same time that Newscom was taking this action in San Francisco, he joined with Anderson and R. T. Rybak, the mayor of Minneapolis, to sponsor a resolution at the U.S. Conference of Mayors in Los Angeles to "encourage a compilation of information regarding the importance of municipal water and the impact of bottled water on municipal waste."[26] Although representatives from Coco-Cola and the American Beverage Association spoke against the resolution, it passed.

Anti-bottled water actions have been taken in other places as well. With its water coming from the Catskills, New York City began an advertising campaign to encourage residents to drink "cool, healthy, clean . . . NYC water."[27] The Berkeley, California, school district replaced machines that contained bottled water with containers of tap water. A 2007 article in *The New York Times* notes that Ann Cooper, the director of the district's nutrition services said, "The students were up in arms, but a year later no one says anything. We have been marketed to the point that children believe they can't drink water out of the tap."[28]

Other cities in California, including Emeryville, Los Angeles, Santa Barbara, and San Leandro, have told their city departments not to purchase bottled water or have discontinued bottled water contracts. The midwestern city of Ann Arbor, Michigan, has taken similar action.[29]

Individual restaurants are also taking a stand against bottled water. Famed chef Alice Waters, of the Berkeley, California, restaurant Chez Panisse, banished bottled water from the menu in the spring of 2007. Shortly thereafter, Mario Batali, from the *Food Network*, removed bottled water from his Manhattan restaurants, including the upscale Del Posto. Even neighborhood restaurants, such as the Bella Luna in the Jamaica Plain section of Boston and the Farmers Diner in Quechee, Vermont, have no bottled water.[30] In addition, in 2007 the eight-unit Big Bowl chain, which is owned by Lettuce Entertain You Enterprises Inc. and located in Chicago, Minneapolis, and Reston, Virginia, decided it would stop offering bottled water. The company expected that this action would result in annual losses of $25,000.[31]

Some colleges and universities are also encouraging students to drink tap water. The University of Maryland has two water-filtration stations on campus, and students are asked to use these to fill their reusable bottles or glasses. Bottled water is no longer offered in the dining halls. Moreover, a Cathy Guisewite "Cathy" comic strip that described the negative environmental impact of bottled water has been placed near the water stations in every dining hall.[32] Similarly, at Bowdoin College in Brunswick, Maine, students drink filtered tap water. Often, students may be seen filling their reusable mugs.[33]

A few organizations have emerged to help raise public awareness about the negative aspects of bottled water and the need to support the maintenance of public water systems. One such group is the Washington, D.C.-based Food & Water Watch. In its article length publication, "Take Back the Tap," Food & Water Watch explains that Aquafina (purified tap water) registered $425.7 million in sales in 2005. During that same year, Dasani (also purified tap water) brought in $346.1 million. So, bottled water cost consumers 240 to 10,000 times more per gallon than tap water. "In many cases, consumers are spending all that extra money . . . because they have bought into the beverage industry's marketing magic that water in a plastic bottle is safer and healthier than tap water."[34]

At the same time, "Take Back the Tap" contends that the FDA has "a woeful record of protecting consumer health and safety." And it has devoted "less than one full-time employee . . . to bottled water oversight."[35]

Another group, Think Outside the Bottle, was formed by Corporate Accountability International (formerly Infact), which has a history of taking on corporate giants. Think Outside the Bottle is a "collective effort of major national organizations, cities, prominent people, communities of faith, student groups, and concerned consumers across North America" who want to encourage people to select tap water over bottled water.[36] To this group, even recycling water bottles is not acceptable. It also uses a huge amount of energy. "To visualize the entire energy costs of the lifecycle of a bottle of water, imagine filling up a quarter of each bottle with oil."[37]

According to a 2008 article in E, the mystique that once surrounded bottled water is over. "These days, it's the tap water enthusiasts, concerned about the environment, who get to act self-righteous. Just like it has become cool to bring your own cloth bags to the grocery store and your own mug to the coffee shop, the reusable water bottle is the nip, new ecoaccessory."[38]

It is not surprising that the bottled water industry has been fighting efforts to diminish their enormous share of the water market. The International Bottled Water Association (IBWA) maintains that bottled water should not be pitted against public drinking water systems. Rather, most people drink both bottled water and tap water. As a result, in an article published in 2007, the organization noted that it is concerned with "strengthening, not undermining, municipal water sources and bottled water sales have nothing to do with tap water infrastructure funding or drinking water system improvements."[39] According to Joseph Doss, IBWA president and CEO, "Drinking water is good. If it's tap water, it's good; if it's bottled water, it's good."[40]

In another article published in 2007, the IBWA noted that when discussing the impact of plastic on the environment it was unfair to single out the bottled water industry, which represents only a "small portion of the packaged beverage category." Instead, there should be an increased focus on encouraging all forms of package recycling. "Any other approach misses a real opportunity to arrive at a comprehensive solution to protecting and sustaining the environment."[41] To help spread the word about the safety of bottled and aggressive recycling practices, in August 2007 the IBWA ran full-page ads in *The New York Times* and *The San Francisco Chronicle*.

Based near Reykjavik, Iceland, Icelandic Water Holdings contends that it has found a solution to the environmental problems associated with bottled water. It primarily uses nonpolluting geothermal (derived from Iceland's underground volcanic activity) power to pump and bottle its water. As a result, the company maintains that its water is "carbon neutral—meaning it has eliminated any contribution to global warming."[42] Icelandic Water Holdings also purchased "'carbon offsets' to abate the environmental effects of its shipping activity." For the year ending in March 2008, it paid for 552 tons of emissions. A paid consulting firm even issued the company a carbon-neutral certification.[43]

However, a 2007 article in *BusinessWeek* commented that Icelandic Water Holdings purchased too few carbon offsets. Five hundred fifty-two offsets are equal to the emissions from twenty-three Americans over the course of one year. "How can that suffice for a company that ships millions of bottles of water, weighing eight pounds per gallon, for distances up to 4,300 miles?"[44] Then again, the article continued, Icelandic Water Holdings is not accounting for the distribution of the water after it arrives at its destination, which in the United States is Richmond, Virginia. "Trucking, in particular, generates lots of carbon for which Icelandic simply isn't accounting."[45]

Four weeks after the article appeared, *BusinessWeek* printed a letter from Patrick Racz, the CEO of Icelandic Water Holdings. In his note, Racz said that the article's author presented an inaccurate assessment of his company. For example, the author failed to mention that Icelandic's carbon imprint is "one-third lower than the industry average" and that it is the only bottled water company to have a carbon-neutral certification, requiring a strict certification process. Racz said that *BusinessWeek*'s failure to publish the "full facts" sends a poor message to other bottling companies that may be trying to "make positive environmental changes."[46]

Bottled water is also being used to help raise money for charities, medical problems, and the needs of people living in Third World countries. One of the most successful is Athena Partners, which sells bottled water to raise money for research on breast and gynecological cancers. The company, which was incorporated in December 2002, was the brainchild of Trish May, a former marketing executive at Microsoft. When she retired from Microsoft in 1999, she had savings from her six-figure salary and a stock options package. In reality, she would never need to work again. And, yet, after battling breast cancer and losing her mother to ovarian cancer, May used over $500,000 of her own money to form Athena Partners. A 2007 article in *U. S. News & World Report* notes that the water "is purified tap water with added minerals, similar to Coca-Cola's Dasani." It has been estimated that the company sold 14 million bottles in 2007; revenues were $2.5 million, up 25 percent from 2006.[47] After taxes, 100 percent of the net profits are donated; and, though she works long hours, May earns no salary.

Meanwhile, in 2001, while working as business consultant in South Africa, Peter Thum saw that many people did not have access to clean water or sanitation services. As a result, together with Jonathan Greenblatt, a friend and business school classmate, he created a business, Ethos Water. According to the business plan, part of the profits of each bottle would be donated to clean water initiatives in Third World countries, and the Ethos Water social message would be written on each bottle. After several years of struggle, Thum and Greenblatt's big break came when they were able to spread the word about their water at an annual technology, entertainment, and design conference in Monterey, California. According to Thum, the partners "arranged for our bottles to be placed inside the gift bags handed out to guests." And they "built displays near each door with posters featuring children from the projects we had funded."[48] In fact, they made Ethos Water so ubiquitous that they "feared being kicked out."[49]

But that didn't happen. Instead, Pierre Omidyar, the founder of eBay, stopped at their table to talk and discuss Ethos Water. It was Omidyar who introduced Thum and Greenblatt to Howard Schultz, the founder of Starbucks. In 2005 Ethos Water was sold to Starbucks for $7.7 million. By the year 2010 the company hopes to donate more than $10 million a year to nonprofit groups that fund safe water projects.[50]

But is that a reasonable projection? It is not entirely clear. In the previously noted book *Bottlemania*, Elizabeth Royte notes that, "a nickel for every bottle, up to $10 million over five years, goes to nonprofits that focus on water delivery, sanitation, and hygiene. To reach the goal of $10 million, Starbucks will have to sell forty million bottles of water a year—water trucked from springs in Baxter, California, and Hazleton, Pennsylvania—leaving behind $350 million in revenue when all is said and done."[51]

Royte adds that while ethical waters enables consumers to feel good about their purchases, they still have negative side effects. "They undermine confidence in tap water, which may erode public support that crucial for its upkeep and improvement; they do nothing to solve the problems that spur consumers to buy bottled water in the first place; they perpetuate the idea that water is a commodity; and they subtly make us forget that Starbucks, or any other food-service establishment, has a perfectly good spigot behind its counter."[52]

It is important to mention that water companies are beginning to reduce their environmental impact. In a 2007 article authored by Kim

Jeffrey, the president and CEO of Nestlé Waters North America, the producer of Poland Spring, Perrier, Arrowhead, Ice Mountain, San Pellegrino, and Deer Park, Jeffrey notes that Nestlé Waters has created the ultralight Eco-Shape bottle. With an average weight of 12.5 grams, it is, according to Jeffrey, "the lightest half-liter bottle in beverage industry history." Because it uses one-third fewer plastic than the other half-liter containers, only 12 ounces of plastic are needed to produce each case of water.[53]

Another 2007 article that appeared in *Beverage World* noted that David DeCecco, a spokesman for PepsiCo, said that since 2002, his company "reduced the weight of its 500 ml Aquafina bottle nearly 40 percent, from 24 to 15 grams," and "the weight of its 20-ounce bottle nearly 15 percent."[54]

The same article notes that Scott Vitters, the director of sustainable packaging for Coca-Cola, said that in 2007 his company reduced the amount of plastic that it uses by about 10 percent. This was accomplished "through packaging redesign efforts and light weighting initiatives."[55]

So, which is better—bottled or tap? In most instances, tap water is just fine. For those who are unsure of the status of their tap water, it is relatively easy to check with local water departments. Representatives of the water department are able to provide information about the quality of the water. They can also issue copies of the Annual Water Quality Report, also known as Consumer Confidence Report. Water representatives may also direct residents to local water testing laboratories and facilities.

In the relatively uncommon instances when the tap water should not be consumed, a simple water filter placed on the kitchen faucet will probably provide all the filtering that most people require. Different water filters are used for the various contaminants. If the water is truly terrible, consider a whole—house filtration system. But these are obviously more expensive to install and maintain. Of course, when away from home, bottled water might be easier to manage. And, in the end, they should be recycled. Or, better yet, use stainless steel or lined aluminum bottles.

Finally, though it may not work in every state, there is the potential for the expansion of the bottle return laws. In a number of states, when people purchase certain types of bottles, they are charged a deposit. When these bottles are returned, so are the deposits. While the amounts may be relatively small, some individuals will have a greater incentive to return their bottles, and some others may make effort to collect those carelessly thrown by others.

CONCLUSION

Years ago, one rarely saw people walking around with bottled water. Just about always, water was obtained from the faucet. And servers in restaurants almost never asked if patrons wanted bottled water. Today, bottled water is a massive, multibillion dollar industry. But it is a industry heavily dependent upon oil, at a time when there is concern about the cost of oil and the ever-growing threat of global warming. While it remains an individual decision whether to purchase bottled water, those who do decide to use bottled water should recycle them and, when appropriate, support bottle return laws.

TOPICS FOR DISCUSSION

1. Do you drink bottled water? Why or why not?
2. Did reading this chapter change your opinion about drinking bottled water? Explain.
3. Do you believe that bottled water is worth the extra cost? Why or why not?
4. In the past, have you recycled your bottles? Has reading this chapter changed how you feel about recycling? Why or why not?
5. Before reading this article, did you know that bottled water could actually be tap water? Has that changed how you feel about bottled water?

NOTES

1. Bill Marsh, "A Battle between the Bottle and the Faucet," *The New York Times* (July 15, 2007) IL.

2. International Bottled Water Association website, http://www.bottled water.org, and Bryan Walsh, "Back to the Tap," *Time* (August 20, 2007) 170: 56.

3. "Bottled Water and Snake Oil," *Global Agenda* (July 31, 2007).

4. Adam Voiland, "How Safe Is Your Drinking Water?" *U.S. News & World Report* (July 19, 2007) NA.

5. Francis H. Chapelle, *Wellsprings: A Natural History of Bottled Spring Waters* (New Brunswick, New Jersey: Rutgers University Press, 2005).

6. Elizabeth Royte, *Bottlemania* (New York City: Bloomsburg, 2008) 17.

7. David Lazarus, "Spin the Water Bottle: With $11 Billion in Sales, the Beverage's Marketers Have Become Clear Winners," *San Francisco Chronicle* (January 17, 2007) C-1.

8. Container Recycling Institute website, http://www.container-recycling.org.

9. Worldwatch Institute website, http://www.worldwatch.org.

10. Container Recycling Institute website, http://www.container-recycling.org.

11. Bryan Walsh, "Back to the Tap," *Time* (August 20, 2007) 170: 56.

12. National Association for PET Container Resources website, http://www.napcor.com.

13. Adam Voiland, "The Safety of PET Bottles," *U.S. News & World Report* (July 26, 2007) and press release from the University of Heidelberg.

14. National Resources Defense Council website, http://www.nrdc.org.

15. "Are Consumers Daft Spotlight on Bottled Water," *The Economist (US)* (August 4, 2007) 384: 15.

16. National Resources Defense Council website.

17. National Resources Defense Council website.

18. National Resources Defense Council website.

19. Bill Wolpin "Bottled Watergate," *American City & Country* (August 1, 2007) 122: NA.

20. National Resources Defense Council website.

21. Environmental Working Group website, http://www.ewg.org.

22. Environmental Working Group website.

23. Environmental Working Group website.

24. Michael Blanding, "The Bottled Water Backlash" (October 19, 2007), www.alternet.org/story/65520.

25. Tim Lang, "The True Cost of Bottling Water: Bottled Water May Be Trendy, but It's also Ecologically Stupid. San Francisco's Ban on Buying It Is in Place, but Could It Work Here?" *Grocer* (July 14, 2007) 230: 23.

26. The U.S. Conference of Mayors website, usmayors.org.

27. Michael Blanding, "The Bottled Water Backlash."

28. Marian Burros, "Fighting the Tide, A Few Restaurants Tilt to Tap Water," *The New York Times* (May 30, 2007) F1.

29. Michael Blanding, "The Bottled Water Backlash."

30. Marian Burros, Marian, "Fighting the Tide, A Few Restaurants Tilt to Tap Water."

31. "LEYE's Big Bowl Chain Mixes Bottled Water," *Nation's Restaurant News* (September 3, 2007) 41: 20.

32. E & P Staff, "'Cathy' Comic Helps University's Campaign against Bottled Water," *Editor & Publisher* (September 12, 2007) NA.

33. "Tap Watershed," *Restaurants and Institutions* (October 1, 2007) 117: 12.

34. "Take Back the Tap," Food & Water Watch website (June 2007), 1-2.

35. "Take Back the Tap," Food & Water Watch website, 4.

36. Think Outside the Bottle website, thinkoutsidethebottle.org.

37. Think Outside the Bottle website, thinkoutsidethebottle.org.

38. Melissa Knopper, Melissa, "Backlash." *E* (May—June 2008) 19: 37–39.

39. "Bottled Water Association Launches PR Campaign," *Water World* (September 2007) 23: 112.

40. "Bottled Water Industry Efforts Counter Criticism," *PR Week (US)* (June 6, 2007) 1.

41. "IBWA Defends Water Industry," *Beverage Industry* (August 2007) 98: 12.

42. Ben Elgin, "How 'Green' Is That Water? A Close Look at One Company's Claims of 'Carbon Neutrality' Points to Problems for the Industry," *BusinessWeek* (August 13, 2007) 4046: 68.

43. Ben Elgin, "How 'Green' Is That Water? A Close Look at One Company's Claims of 'Carbon Neutrality' Points to Problems for the Industry."

44. Ben Elgin, "How 'Green' Is That Water? A Close Look at One Company's Claims of 'Carbon Neutrality' Points to Problems for the Industry."

45. Ben Elgin, "How 'Green' Is That Water? A Close Look at One Company's Claims of 'Carbon Neutrality' Points to Problems for the Industry."

46. "Bottled Water and the Environment," *BusinessWeek* (September 10, 2007) 4049: 19.

47. Kerry Hannon, Kerry. "Bottling a Healthy Idea: A Former Microsoft Exec's Start-Up Finances Cancer Research," *U. S. News & World Report* (October 8, 2007) 143: 54.

48. "Ethics in a Bottle," *FSB* (November 2007) 17: 44.

49. "Ethics in a Bottle," 44.

50. "Ethics in a Bottle," 44.

51. Elizabeth Royte, *Bottlemania* (New York City: Bloomsbury, 2008) 162.

52. Elizabeth Royte, *Bottlemania*, 164.

53. Kim Jeffrey, "Water World," *Beverage World* (October 15, 2007) 126: 31.

54. Andrew Kaplan, "How Low Can You Go? Beverage Companies Are Finding That Less Is Often More When It Comes to Packaging," *Beverage World* (October 15, 2007) 126: 51–53.

55. Andrew Kaplan, "How Low Can You Go? Beverage Companies Are Finding That Less Is Often More When It Comes to Packaging."

REFERENCES AND RESOURCES

Books

Bakalar, Nicolas. *Where The Germs Are.* Hoboken, New Jersey: John Wiley & Sons, 2003.

Chapelle, Francis H. *Wellsprings: A Natural History of Bottled Spring Waters.* New Brunswick, New Jersey: Rutgers University Press, 2005.

Royte, Elizabeth. *Bottlemania.* New York City: Bloomsbury, 2008.

Magazines, Journals, and Newspapers

"Are Consumers Daft? Spotlight on Bottled Water." *The Economist (US)* (August 4, 2007) 384: 15.

Blanding, Michael. "The Bottled Water Backlash" (October 19, 2007), www.alternet.org/story/65520.

"Bottled Water and Snake Oil." *Global Agenda* (July 31, 2007).

"Bottled Water and The Environment." *BusinessWeek* (September 10, 2007).

"Bottled Water Association Launches PR Campaign." *Water World* (September 2007) 23: 112.

"Bottled Water Industry Efforts Counter Criticism." *PR Week (US)* (June 6, 2007) 1.

"Bottled Water Sparks Debate." *Cheers* (September 2007) 18: 9.

Burros, Marian. "Fighting the Tide, A Few Restaurants Tilt to Tap Water." *The New York Times* (May 30, 2007) F1.

Crow, Patrick. "Bottled Water Consumption Growing." *Water World* (June 2007) 23: 9.

E & P Staff, "'Cathy' Comic Helps University Campaign Against Bottled Water." *Editor & Publisher* (September 12, 2007).

Elgin, Ben. "How 'Green' Is that Water? A Close Look at One Company's Claims of 'Carbon Neutrality' Points to Problems for the Industry." *BusinessWeek* (August 13, 2007) 4046: 68.

"Ethics in a Bottle." *FSB* (November 2007) 17: 44.

Hannon, Kerry. "Bottling a Healthy Idea: A Former Microsoft Exec's Start-Up Finances Cancer Research." *U. S. News & World Report* (October 8, 2007) 143: 54.

"IBWA Defends Water Industry." *Beverage Industry* (August 2007) 98: 12.

Jeffrey, Kim. "Water World." *Beverage World* (October 15, 2007), 126: 31.

Kaplan, Andrew. "How Low Can You Go? Beverage Companies are Finding That Less Is Often More When it Comes to Packaging." *Beverage World* (October 15, 2007) 126: 51.

Knopper, Melissa. "Backlash." *E Magazine* (May—June 2008) 19: 37–39.

Lang, Tim. "The True Cost of Bottling Water: Bottled Water May Be Trendy, but It's also Ecologically Stupid. San Francisco's Ban on Buying It, but Could It Work Here?" *Grocer* (July 14, 2007) 230: 23.

Lazarus, David. "Spin the (Water) Bottle: With $11 billion in U.S. Sales, the Beverage's Marketers Have Become Clear Winners." *San Francisco Chronicle* (January 17, 2007) C-1.

"LEYE's (Lettuce Entertain You Enterprises Inc.) Big Bowl Nixes Bottled Water." *Nation's Restaurant News* (September 3, 2007) 41: 20.

Marsh, Bill. "A Battle Between the Bottle and the Faucet." *The New York Times* (July 15, 2007) IL.

Matsumoto, Nancy. "Banned!" *People Weekly* (July 16, 2007) 68: 94.

McGowan, Joe. "The Bottle." *Time for Kids* (September 7, 2007) 13: 7.

"Take Back the Tap." Food & Water Watch website (June 2007).

"Tap Watershed." *Restaurants & Institutions* (October 1, 2007) 117: 12.

Todd, Heather. "Saving the World … One Bottle at a Time: Bottled Water Companies Are Donating Profits to Worthy Causes." *Beverage World* (December 15, 2003) 122: 14.

Voiland, Adam. "How Safe is Your Drinking Water?" *U.S. News & World Report* (July 19, 2007), NA.

Voiland, Adam. "The Safety of PET Bottles." *U.S. News & World Report* (July 26, 2007) NA.

Walsh, Bryan. "Back to the Tap." *Time* (August 20, 2007) 170: 56.

"Watershed." *Restaurants & Institutions* (October 1, 2007) 117: 12.

Wopin, Bill. "Bottled Watergate." *American City & County* (August 1, 2007) 122: NA.

Websites

American Water Works Association
http://www.awwa.org

Athena Partners
http://www.athenapartners.org

Container Recycling Institute
http://www.container-recycling.org

Environmental Working Group
http://www.ewg.org

Ethos Water
http://ethoswater.com

Food & Water Watch
http://www.foodandwaterwatch.org

International Bottled Water Association (IBWA)
http://www.bottledwater.org

National Association for PET Container Resources
http://www.napcor.com

National Resources Defense Council
http://www.nrdc.org

The U.S. Conference of Mayors
http://usmayors.org

Think Outside the Bottle
http://thinkoutsidethebottle.org

Worldwatch Institute
http://www.worldwatch.org

Chapter 3

Fast Food

Today, people tend to lead very busy lives. Most people have little extra time for food preparation. So it is very tempting and convenient to consume fast food. And fast food restaurants are ubiquitous. In some urban areas, there may be several on the same block.

A 2007 article in *JOPERD—The Journal of Physical Education, Recreation & Dance*—reports that researchers have estimated that Americans spend over $150 billion a year at the 280,000 fast food restaurants in the United States.[1] Fast food restaurants market heavily to children and adolescents, and for parents pressed for time, it is all too easy just to give into the wishes of their children. Moreover, many fast foods restaurants purposely locate near high schools. That enables teens to eat there frequently, even daily.

This is horrendously problematic. Fast food restaurants are known for serving food that is generally high in fat and calories, and the portions tend to be large. In fact, a study published in 2007 in the *Journal of the American Dietetic Association* seems to indicate that children who regularly eat in fast food restaurants tend to prefer larger portions of French fries, meats, and potato chips and smaller portions of vegetables.[2]

That is exactly what most Americans don't need. Two-thirds of the U.S. population is already overweight; an astonishing one-third of the population is obese. Many of these are children and adolescents. A 2002 article in *The Lancet* notes that the numbers of overweight and obese children "have increased 2.3-fold to 3.3-fold over about 25 years in the USA." Moreover, during this time, the heaviest children have become even heavier. Because minority children are twice as likely as white children to be overweight or obese "pre-existing racial-ethnic disparities" are just made even more difficult.[3] The problem is particularly acute among African-American youth. According to a 2008 article in *Ebony*, "In some U.S. cities, childhood type 2 diabetes has increased

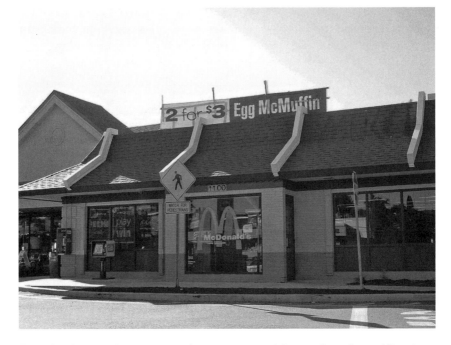

Fast foods may have excessive amounts of fat and sodium. (Courtesy of Mark A. Goldstein)

fivefold in the last decade, with overweight African-American adolescents accounting for nearly 90 percent of the new cases. In fact, the CDC (Centers for Disease Control and Prevention) predicts that if the problem persists, half of the African-American children who were born in 2004 will develop diabetes during their lifetime."[4]

Like adults, children and adolescents who carry so much excess weight are at increased risk for a number of medical problems. The same article in *The Lancet* discusses some of the illnesses that tend to arise in children and adolescents who are overweight or obese. In addition to type 2 diabetes, these are high blood pressure (hypertension), chronic inflammation, increased blood clotting tendency, asymptomatic coronary atherosclerosis, sleep-disordered breathings, asthma, exercise intolerance, hepatic, renal, musculoskeletal, and neurological complications. Moreover, children and adolescents who are overweight or obese have an increased risk for psychological problems. It is not surprising that they frequently develop a negative self-image, and "obese adolescents show declining degrees of self-esteem associated with sadness, loneliness, nervousness, and high-risk behaviors."[5]

A 2004 article published in *Pediatrics* noted that children and adolescents who eat fast food "consumed more total and saturated fat, more total carbohydrate and added sugars, less dietary fiber, and more energy per gram of solid food." They tend to drink sugar-sweetened beverages instead of milk and to eat fewer fruits and nonstarchy vegetables. Furthermore, when children and adolescents eat unhealthful fast foods, they are eating them instead of more healthful alternatives, such as fruits and nonstarchy vegetables.[6]

A study published in 2005 in *The Lancet* examined the relationship between fast food consumption and obesity and type 2 diabetes. The study included black and white men and women between the ages of eighteen and thirty. Researchers found that white women frequented fast food restaurants an average of 1.3 times per week. Black men and women and white men ate fast food an average of twice a week. They also observed that "fast food consumption has strong positive associations with weight gain and insulin resistance, suggesting that fast food increase the risk of obesity and type 2 diabetes."[7]

A study published in 2005 in *Pediatrics* reviewed a cohort of 7,745 girls and 6,610 boys between the ages of nine and fourteen years. Researchers obtained body mass indexes from self-reported heights and weights as well as measures of diet quality and the amount of weekly servings of fried foods away from home (FFA). The findings were not surprising. "Older children who consume greater quantities of FFA are heavier, have greater total energy intakes, and have poor diet quality. Furthermore, increasing consumption of FFA over time may lead to excess weight gain."[8]

Since people throughout the world eat at McDonald's, it may be useful to review the calories, fat, and sodium in some of their products:[9]

Even the most basic foods served at fast food restaurants, such as simple hamburgers, may have higher amounts of sodium. Because most people are advised to consume no more than 2,400 milligrams of sodium (older people or those with cardiovascular problems usually

Food Item	Serving Size (oz)	Calories	Total Fat (g)	Sodium (mg)
Hamburger	3.5	250	9	520
Double Cheeseburger	5.8	440	23	1150
Big Mac	7.5	540	29	1040
Filet-O-Fish	5	380	18	640
McChicken	5	360	16	830
Egg McMuffin	4.8	300	12	820
Sausage Burrito	3.9	300	16	830
Sausage McGriddles	7.1	420	22	1030
Scrambled Eggs (2)	3.3	170	11	180
Hash Browns	2	150	9	340

should consume less), when eating fast food, it is very easy to exceed that amount. In many instances, there are also excessively high levels of fat. A study published in 2007 in the *Journal of Nutrition* described how researchers twice fed participants either a breakfast from McDonald's containing 42 grams of fat or a low-fat meal containing only 1 gram of fat. Researchers found that the "systolic blood pressure, diastolic blood pressure, and total peripheral resistance were greater in participants following the consumption of the high-fat meal relative to the low-fat meal." Thus, "even a single high-fat meal may be associated with heightened cardiovascular reactivity to stress and offer insight into the pathways through which a high-fat diet may affect cardiovascular function."[10]

How about a simple lunch, consisting of a soup, salad, and sandwich from Boston Market? A six-ounce serving of chicken tortilla soup with toppings has 340 calories. Of these, 200 are fat calories, and the soup contains 1,310 milligrams of salt. The caesar side salad, which is only five ounces, has 400 calories. Of these, 360 are fat calories. The salad has 980 milligrams of sodium. The twelve-ounce roasted sirloin open-faced sandwich has 410 calories. Of these, 140 are fat calories, and the sandwich has 1,640 milligrams of salt.[11]

Even more shocking is to read a list of the ingredients in some of the foods. The following are the ingredients contained in the caesar side salad: caesar dressing (soybean oil, water, parmesan cheese [milk, cheese cultures, salt, enzymes], red wine vinegar, egg yolk, salt, lemon juice concentrate, sugar, spices (including mustard seed), anchovy, dehydrated garlic, dehydrated worcestershire sauce [vinegar, corn syrup, salt, spices, dehydrated garlic, tamarind, natural flavor], xanthan gum, dehydrated onion), romaine lettuce, three cheese blend (parmesan, asiago, and romano [milk, cheese cultures, salt, enzymes, and anti-caking agent]), buttery garlic croutons (enriched flour [wheat flour, malted barley flour, niacin, reduced iron, thiamine mononitrate, riboflavin, folic acid], partially hydrogenated soybean oil, maltodextrins, corn syrup, salt, contains 2% or less of each of the following: garlic powder, yeast, corn meal, calcium sulfate, autolyzed yeast, calcium propionate (preservative), dehydrated parsley, natural flavor and color, spice tocopherols (antioxidants), enzymes). Contains: wheat, soy, milk, egg, fish.[12] To even the casual observer, there seem to be too many ingredients with too many strange sounding names.

Researchers at the Center for Science in the Public Interest wondered whether ingredient lists were readily available in fast food restaurants. So, in August 2004, they visited twenty-nine of the thirty-three (88 percent) McDonald's outlets in Washington, D.C. In addition to inspecting the interior space of the outlets, they asked cashiers and restaurant manager to point out nutrition information. "In Washington, DC, 59% of McDonald's outlets provided in-store nutrition information for the majority of their standard menu items. In 62% of the restaurants, it was necessary to ask two or more employees in order to obtain a copy of that information." As a result, the researchers concluded that even in the largest fast food chain in the United States, "nutrition information at the point of decision-making is often difficult to find or completely absent."[13]

A 2008 article in *Obesity Reviews* notes that all too many foods sold at fast food restaurants contain "unacceptably high levels of industrially produced trans fatty acids." (See chapter 4.) Trans fatty acids, which have only a negative impact on the body, "contribute to type 2 diabetes and coronary artery disease." Furthermore, there is now good evidence that trans fatty acids support abdominal obesity, "an important factor in the metabolic syndrome, type 2 diabetes, and cardiovascular disease."[14]

In his book *The Fast Food Diet*, which was published in 2006, Stephen Sinatra, a cardiologist, maintains that people can, indeed, include fast food in their diets. Sinatra believes in the 80/20 Rule. If people eat truly healthfully 80 percent of the time, "it's okay to splurge the other 20 percent." Sinatra contends that most diets fail because they are too rigid. "They may work for a week or two, but sooner or later everyone gets tired of following the rules—and, rebels that we are, we break them. But the 80/20 Rule is one you can follow for life, because it gives you room to take a break."[15] Moreover, Sinatra says that all fast food is not unhealthful. "There are quite a few menu items that are highly nutritious and modest in calories."[16] For example, at Arby's, a good choice is the regular roast beef sandwich. It has 320 calories, thirteen grams of total fat, and six grams of saturated fat. "For most folks, one is all it takes—and it's lean enough to have every day."[17] While many of the items on Burger King's menu are too high in calories and the portions are too large, Fire-Grilled Chicken and Shrimp Garden Salad each have 310 calories, eighteen grams total fat, and four grams saturated fat. "This flavorful meat-and-garden salad is filling enough for a full meal, and healthy enough to enjoy without worrying about calories. If you get it with shrimp, you'll also give yourself a blast of those healthy omega-3 fatty acids."[18]

The Subway restaurants seem to have a number of different healthful choices. One of Sinatra's favorites is the Sweet Onion Chicken Teriyaki Sandwich (six-inch), which has 380 calories, five grams of total fat, and 1.5 grams of saturated fat. "I love the onions on this sandwich—not just because I'm an onion lover, but because onions contain some of the most healthful plant chemicals ever discovered—chemicals that protect the cardiovascular system and, along with other vegetables, help prevent heart attacks." Another good choice is the six-inch Veggie Delite Sandwich, which as 230 calories, three grams total fat, and one gram saturated fat. "You could eat this sandwich every day for the rest of your life and keep your weight right where you want it."[19]

Sinatra offers a number of general suggestions for eating in fast food restaurants: Chicken without the skin tends to be lower in calories than hamburgers. Don't eat the French fries, which contain far too much fat and may well contain trans fat. A roast beef sandwich is normally leaner than a hamburger. Eat smaller amounts of cheese, which is almost entirely fat. Avoid the "special meals," which tend to be high in calories. Enjoy the salads, but limit the salad dressings. Add toppings, such as tomatoes, onions, lettuce, green peppers, and cucumbers. Stay away from the sodas, which are empty calories.[20]

In *Guide to Health Fast-Food Eating*, which was published by the American Dietetic Association in 2006, Hope S. Warshaw lists ten suggestions for "eating out healthfully." First, while eating out, diners should have a "can do" attitude. Instead of equating eating out with "pigging out," diners should believe that they are able to eat healthfully when they eat outside the home. Second, people who eat large numbers of meals outside the home should find ways to change this habit and eat more of their meals at home.

Third, search for restaurants that offer better options. Fourth, even before entering the restaurants diners should "envision a healthy and enjoyable outcome." It is important not to "become a victim of hasty choices or be swayed by the sights and smells." Fifth, diners must become "well-trained fat detectors" and avoid foods containing high amounts of fat such as butter, mayonnaise-base sauces, sausage, and bacon.

Sixth, diners should always eat what falls within their food plan. "Try to fulfill each food group requirement with menu items, or substitute foods to make your meal complete." Seventh, eat reasonable portions. "Take advantage of smaller serving sizes, and don't get taken in by meal deal or more food for less money come-ons." Eight, people should practice a little creativity with their dining. "Consider, for example, splitting a sandwich or salad with your dining partner." Ninth, diners should feel free to ask for foods to be made to order. For example, instead of eating a sandwich made with a croissant, diners should request whole wheat bread. Finally, diners should know that they do not need to eat everything on their plate. "To keep from overeating, don't order too much, order creatively, and push your plate away when you meet your calories needs."[21]

Warshaw also offers a numbers of suggestions for selecting better choices in specific types of fast food restaurants. For example, in chicken chains, diners should remove the skin. If the meal is large, divide it into two portions. The second portion may be taken home. Because the white meat is lower in fat, whenever there is a choice, select white meat. It is best to order à la carte and pick side dishes such as corn and beans. Avoid the biscuits and hushpuppies.[22] And, how about eating at pizza chains? Warshaw says that it is best to order lots of healthier toppings such as part-skim cheese, sliced tomatoes, green peppers, onions, broccoli, and mushrooms. Limit the amount of not-so-healthy toppings such as extra cheese, anchovies, pepperoni, bacon, and sausage.[23]

In the 2008 book *Eat This Not That!* written by David Zinczenko with Matt Goulding, the authors give exact suggestions on what to eat and what not to eat in a number of different fast food restaurants. The photo and fact-filled book is fairly small in size; the authors intend for people to take the book along when visiting fast food establishments. In fact, the authors state that they want readers to *use* the book. "Use it when you're out with friends. Use it when you're shopping for your family. Use it when you're idling in the drive-thru, waiting to talk to a clown. Use it to make smart, health, fat-busting food choices no matter where you are."[24]

So, for example, when purchasing food at the Boston Market chain of stores, Zinczenko and Goulding advise eating roast sirloin, garlic dill, new potatoes, and spinach. This option has 560 calories, twenty-seven grams of fat, and 760 milligrams of sodium. At the same time, the authors suggest that their readers not eat the meal that contains three pieces of dark chicken, sweet potatoes, and Market Chopped Side Salad. Such a meal has 1,410 calories, ninety grams of fat, and 3,020 milligrams of sodium. They note that the salad is "a fatty blend of soybean oil, white whine vinegar, Dijon mustard, and honey. A single serving has thirty-nine grams of fat."[25]

CONCLUSION

With people leading such busy lives, it is very easy to save time on food preparation by eating a diet that includes lots of fast foods. Unfortunately, the majority of fast foods are high in calories and salt. But there are fast food options that are lower in calories and salt. When making fast food choices, it is better to try to select those.

TOPICS FOR DISCUSSION

1. What are the advantages and disadvantages of eating fast foods? How often do you eat fast food? Do you think that is too much? Why or why not?

2. Do you have a fast food restaurant in your school? Do you think schools should have fast food restaurants? Why or why not?

3. To help people eat more balanced diets, what additional foods should fast food restaurants offer?

4. Do you believe that there should be regulations that require fast food restaurants to offer healthier options? Why or why not?

5. Do you think that fast food contributes significantly to obesity in teens or adults? Why or why not?

NOTES

1. Nestor W. Shermon, "Children, Schools, and Fast Food," *JOPERD—The Journal of Physical Education, Recreation & Dance* (April 2007) 78(4): 12.

2. Cynthia K. Colapinto, Angela Fitzgerald, L. Janette Taper, and Paul J. Veugelers, "Children's Preference for Large Portions: Prevalence, Determinants, and Consequences," *Journal of the American Dietetic Association* (July 2007) 107(7): 1183–90.

3. Cara B. Ebbeling, Dorota B. Pawlak, and David S. Ludwig, "Childhood Obesity: Public-Health Crisis, Common Sense Cure," *The Lancet* (August 10, 2002) 360(9331): 473.

4. Kevin Chappel, "Black Youths: The New Face of Diabetes: As African-American Youngsters Have Become Heavier, Half of Them Are Predicted To Be Diagnosed with the Disease During Their Lifetime," *Ebony* (March 2008) 63(5): 130–3.

5. Cara B. Ebbeling, Dorota B. Pawlak, and David S. Ludwig, "Childhood Obesity: Public-Health Crisis, Common Sense Cure," *The Lancet* (August 10, 2002) 360(9331): 473.

6. Shanthy A. Bowman, Steven L. Gortmaker, Cara B. Ebbeling, et al., "Effects of Fast-Food Consumption of Energy Intake and Diet Quality among Children in a National Household Survey," *Pediatrics* (January 2004) 113(1): 112–18.

7. Mark A. Pereira, Alex I. Kartashov, Cara B. Ebbeling, et al., "Fast-Food Habits, Weight Gain, and Insulin Resistance (the CARDIA Study): 15-Year Prospective Analysis," *The Lancet* (January 1, 2005) 365(9453): 36.

8. Elsi M. Taveras, Catherine S. Berkey, Sheryl L. Rifas-Shiman, et al., "Association of Consumption of Fried Food Away from Home with Body Mass Index and Diet Quality in Older Children and Adolescents," *Pediatrics* (October 2005) 116(4): 1010.

9. McDonald's Corporation website, http://mcdonalds.com.

10. Fabijana Jakulj, Kristin Zernicke, Simon L. Bacon, et al., "A High-Fat Meal Increases Cardiovascular Reactivity to Psychological Stress in Healthy Young Adults," *Journal of Nutrition* (April 2007) 137(4): 935–9.

11. Boston Market website, http://www.bostonmarket.com.

12. Boston Market website.

13. Margo G. Wooten, Melissa Osborn, and Claudia J. Malloy, "Availability of Point-of-Purchase Nutrition Information at a Fast-Food Restaurant," *Preventive Medicine* (December 2006) 43(6): 458–9.

14. Arne Astrup, Jorn Dyerberg, Matthew Selleck, and Steen Stender, "Nutrition Transition and its Relationship to the Development of Obesity and Related Chronic Diseases," *Obesity Reviews* (March 2008) 9: 48–52.

15. Stephen Sinatra, *The Fast Food Diet* (Hoboken, New Jersey: John Wiley & Sons, Inc., 2006) 11.

16. Stephen Sinatra, *The Fast Food Diet*, 12.

17. Stephen Sinatra, *The Fast Food Diet*, 50.

18. Stephen Sinatra, *The Fast Food Diet*, 52–3.

19. Stephen Sinatra, *The Fast Food Diet*, 59.

20. Stephen Sinatra, *The Fast Food Diet*, 64–6.

21. Hope S. Warshaw, *Guide to Healthy Fast-Food Eating* (Alexander, Virginia: American Dietetic Association, 2006) 15–17.

22. Hope S. Warshaw, *Guide to Healthy Fast-Food Eating*, 39–40.

23. Hope S. Warshaw, *Guide to Healthy Fast-Food Eating*, 41.

24. David Zinczenko, with Matt Goulding, *Eat This Not That!* (New York: Rodale, 2008) vi.

25. David Zinczenko, with Matt Goulding, *Eat This Not That!* , 36–7.

REFERENCES AND RESOURCES

Books

Ludwig, David with Suzanne Rostler. *Ending the Food Flight*. Boston and New York: Houghton Mifflin Company, 2007.

Sinatra, Stephen and Jim Punkre. *The Fast Food Diet*. Hoboken, New Jersey: John Wiley & Sons, Inc., 2006.

Warshaw, Hope S. *Guide to Healthy Fast-Food Eating*. Alexandria, Virginia: American Dietetic Association, 2006.

Zinczenko, David with Matt Goulding. *Eat This Not That!* New York: Rodale, 2008.

Magazines, Journals, and Newspapers

Astrup, Arne, Jorn Dyerberg, Matthew Selleck, and Steen Stender. "Nutrition Transition and its Relationship to the Development of Obesity and Related Chronic Diseases." *Obesity Reviews* (March 2008) 9: 48–52.

Bowman, Shanthy A., Steven L. Gortmaker, Cara B. Ebbeling, et al. "Effects of Fast-Food Consumption on Energy Intake and Diet Quality among Children in a National Household Survey." *Pediatrics* (January 2004) 113(1): 112–18.

Chappel, Kevin. "Black Youths: The New Face of Diabetes: As African-American Youngsters Have Become Heavier, Half of Them Are Predicted To Be Diagnosed with the Disease During Their Lifetime." *Ebony* (March 2008) 63(5): 130–3.

Colapinto, Cynthia K., Angela Fitzgerald, L. Janette Taper, and Paul J. Veugelers. "Children's Preference for Large Portions: Prevalence, Determinants, and Consequences." *Journal of the American Dietetic Association* (July 2007) 107(7): 1183–90.

Ebbeling, Cara B., Dorota B. Pawlak, and David Ludwig. "Childhood Obesity: Public–Health Crisis, Common Sense Cure." *The Lancet* (August 10, 2002) 360(9331): 473.

Ellman, Marc. "Single Fast-Food Meal Increases Blood Pressure." *Life Extension* (August 2007) NA.

Jakulj, Fabijana, Kristin Zernicke, and Simon L. Bacon et al. "A High-Fat Meal Increases Cardiovascular Reactivity to Psychological Stress in Health Young Adults." *Journal of Nutrition* (April 2007) 137(4): 935–9.

Pereira, Mark A., Alex I. Kartashov, Cara B. Ebbeling, et al. "Fast-Food Habits, Weight Gain, and Insulin Resistance (the CARDIA Study): 15-Year Prospective Analysis." *The Lancet* (January 1, 2005) 365(9453): 36.

Sherman, Nestor W. "Children, Schools, and Fast Food." *JOPERD—The Journal of Physical Education, Recreation & Dance* (April 2007) 78(4): 12.

Taveras, Elsie M., Catherine S. Berkey, Sheryl L. Rifas-Shiman et al. "Association of Consumption of Fried Food Away from Home with Body Mass Index and Diet Quality in Older Children and Adolescents." *Pediatrics* (October 2005) 116(4): 1010.

Wootan, Margo G., Melissa Osborn, and Claudia J. Malloy. "Availability of Point-of-Purchase Nutrition Information at a Fast-Food Restaurant." *Preventive Medicine* (December 2006) 43(6): 458–9.

Websites

Boston Market
http://www.bostonmarket.com

McDonald's Corporation
http://mcdonalds.com

Chapter 4

Fats

Historically, fat was considered a very valued food. Those who could include increased amounts of fat in their diets had greater protection from starvation during times of scarcity. Even today, while food is plentiful in the developed world, in many parts of the developing world, people are often unable to consume sufficient amounts of food. For those individuals, carrying a little extra weight is considered far more desirable than being too thin. Women with rounder figures are believed to be more attractive than those who are lean; women with extra poundage are also thought to be more fertile and more likely to give birth to a healthy child.

But this is a chapter about fats in America. By the second half of the twentieth century, Americans tended to loop all fats together—assigning them all negative labels. Americans were told to limit their consumption of all types of fat. Fats were thought to raise the risk for a host of different medical problems, such as heart disease and cancer. Moreover, those who consumed larger amounts of fat tended to become heavier or even obese. After all, excess weight and obesity have become epidemic in the United States.

Yet, in recent years, many people have begun to realize that fats are an integral part of the human body. According to Rosemary Stanton, in *Good Fats Bad Fats*, a book published in 2002, without fat, it is impossible to achieve optimal health. People need fat to regulate body temperature; fat protects the body from extreme heat and cold. Fat provides cushioning for internal organs and padding for bones. Fat stores energy, which is especially important during time of illness. Fat is required to build and support nerve and brain cells, and fat is needed to produce hormones and absorb some nutrients.[1] "We need to stop thinking of all body fat as undesirable. Some is essential."[2]

A 2007 article entitled "Oil is Well" in *Prevention* magazine notes that, "consuming less than 20% of your calories from fats and oils may actually

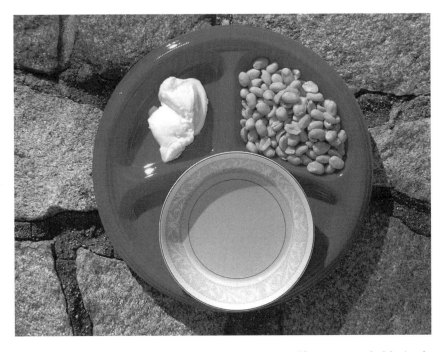

Some fats are healthy and some are not. (Courtesy of Mark A. Goldstein)

increase your risk of heart disease. That's because a deficit can lower your intake of vitamin E (a powerful antioxidant), keep 'good' cholesterol from rising, and spike triglycerides (type of fat found in the body)."[3]

UNSATURATED FATS

There are two types of unsaturated fats that help to lower blood cholesterol: polyunsaturated fats and monounsaturated fats. Unsaturated fats, which are liquid at room temperature, are derived from plant or animal sources.

Polyunsaturated Fats

When consuming fats, it is important to distinguish between those that support good health and those that don't. More than thirty years ago, researchers discovered a class of fats known as polyunsaturated fatty acids (PUFA). There are two main types of polyunsaturated fatty acids: omega-3 and omega-6. Both are essential fatty acids that the body requires but is unable to manufacture. A 2007 article in *Natural Health* explains that, in general, omega-3 fatty acids, which are contained in fish, nuts, and flaxseed, are considered good fats. Most omega-6s, which are found in corn, cottonseed, and soybean oils, margarine, processed foods as well as "the infamous trans fats that come from the partial hydrogenation of vegetable oil," have a negative effect on the body.[4] There does appear to be one member of the omega-6 fatty acids, conjugated linoleic acid (CLA), which is "found only in the meat and milk of ruminants such as cattle,"[5] that is beneficial. There is some evidence that it may help with weight loss, build lean mass, increase immunity, and stop the growth of cancer cells. "The word fat here is crucial: Because CLA is found only in the fat of ruminants and their milk, you won't find it in skim milk or non-fat yogurt."[6] (But new evidence has found CLA in white button mushrooms.)

Omega-3s were once a plentiful part of the American diet. A 2007 article in *Environmental Nutrition* notes "that's because cattle and chickens used to graze on rich sources of omega-3s like grass, wild plants, and seeds, instead of grains with scant omega-3s, which is what agribusiness now typically uses as livestock feed."[7]

A 2006 article in *Women's Health* noted that it is generally agreed that people should consume about 3,000 milligrams per day of omega-6 and 1,000 milligrams of omega-3. "That 3:1 ratio is important: Some studies show that eating too many omega-6s and not enough omega-3s may negate the positive health effects."[8] A 2005 article in the *Saturday Evening Post* says that the "typical American diet tends to contain up to 30 times more omega-6 fatty acids than omega-3 fatty acids."[9] It is this imbalance that is thought to contribute to a host of different medical problems.

One such problem is major depression. A study published in 2007 in *Psychosomatic Medicine* found that the omega-6 to omega-3 ratio in subjects with major depression to be 18 to 1. In subjects without depression, the ratio was 13 to 1. As the ratio rose, so did the degree of severity of the depression.[10] The researchers also found an association between higher levels of omega-6 and inflammation-causing compounds that have been linked to arthritis, type 2 diabetes, and heart disease.

Research published a year earlier in *Brown University Psychopharmacology Update* noted a possible link between suicide and higher omega-6/omega-3 ratios. Researchers studied thirty-three subjects with major depressive disorder. During a two-year follow-up, seven attempted suicide at least once. Two of these attempts were fatal. All of the subjects who attempted suicide had elevated ratios. Commenting on the study, David L. Katz, an associate professor of public health and director of the Prevention Research Center at Yale University School of Medicine, said, "While more research is needed before the use of omega-3 fatty acids can be considered among the routine therapies for depression, our knowledge is certainly sufficient to justify efforts to increase prevailing intake levels. We may hope that by doing so there might be less depression to treat."[11]

In a 2004 population study published in *Lipids,* researchers examined the association between consumption of omega-6 fatty acids and the murder rates in Argentina, Australia, Canada, the United Kingdom, and the United States. It is of interest that the researchers found that in areas where there were higher than average consumption of omega-6 fatty acids, there were also higher than average rates of murder. The rates of homicide appeared to correlate directly with increases in consumption of omega-6 fatty acids. The researchers concluded that, "these dietary interventions merit exploration as relatively cost-effective measures for reducing the pandemic of violence in Western societies, just as dietary interventions are reducing cardiovascular mortality."[12]

A culture stimulated tumor growth laboratory study published in 2005 in *Carcinogenesis* found that reducing the intake of omega-6 lowers the risk for cancer. It is believed that people who have higher intakes of omega-6 increase their risk for prostate cancer.[13] In another article, published in 2005 in *GP*, the lead researcher of the study, Millie Hughes-Fulford, said that people who consume higher amounts of omega-6 are also at increased risk for colorectal and some breast cancers.[14]

A 2004 article in *Women's Health Weekly* describes Spanish researchers at the Universitat Autonoma de Barcelona who induced breast cancer tumors in rats. When the rats were fed excess amounts of omega-6, the tumors grew faster. While omega-6 fatty acids do not cause cancer, they clearly have the potential to "accelerate the clinical development of the disease."[15]

In her book, *The Ultimate Omega-3 Diet*, registered dietician Evelyn Tribole lists the omega-6 content of nuts. (Remember, nuts also contain omega-3 fatty acids.) While nuts are generally believed to be healthful, it may be wise to limit or avoid those with the highest levels of omega-6:[16]

Type of Nut(one ounce or two tablespoons)	Omega-6 Fat(milligrams)
Walnuts	10,800
Sunflower seeds, roasted	9,700
Pine nuts	9,400
Hemp nut seeds	9,400
Pumpkin and squash seeds	5,870
Hickory nuts	5,850
Pecans	5,850
Brazil nuts	5,820
Peanuts	4,450
Pistachio nuts	3,740
Hazelnuts	2,220
Cashews	2,170
Chestnuts	450
Macadamia nuts	370

Tribole also offers a number of food substitutions that may help reduce the amount of omega-6 in the diet. Some of these are as follows: [17]

Instead of	Use
Granola, regular	Flax-based or canola-oil based granola
Peanut butter	Almond butter, cashew butter, macadamia nut butter
Margarine, standard	Canola oil margarine
Eggs	Omega-3 eggs
Potato chips, regular	Baked chips; chips made with olive oil And high-oleic oils
Tuna in oil	Light tuna in water

OMEGA-3

There has been a good deal of research on omega-3s. The vast majority of studies have found that consumption of omega-3s yields positive results. For example, a study published in 2007 in *Hypertension* examined 5,000 adults between the ages of forty and figty-nine who lived in China, Japan, the United Kingdom, and the United States. After the researchers adjusted for variables such as age, weight, gender, salt intake, and exercise, they found that people who ate higher amounts of foods rich in omega-3 fatty acids had lower blood pressure readings than those who ate lower amounts of omega-3 fatty acids. The researchers concluded that omega-3 fatty acids may "contribute to prevention and control of adverse blood pressure levels."[18]

A 2005 article entitled "New Study Shows Fish Oil Supplementation Benefits Arthritic Patients" in *Townsend Letter for Doctors and Patients* describes research conducted by Joseph Maroon and Jeff Bost that was presented before an annual meeting of the American Association of Neurological Surgeons. Patients with nonsurgical neck or back pain were given two types of omega-3s. After seventy-five days of supplementation, 60 percent of the subjects "reported reduction in both overall pain and joint pain, and 59% discontinued taking prescription pain medications or non-steroidal anti-inflammatory drugs (NSAIDs)."[19] Eighty percent of the subjects reported that they were satisfied with their improvement, and 88 percent said that they would continue with the supplementation.[20]

A study published in 2005 in *The American Journal of Clinical Nutrition* reviewed the association between diet and dry eye syndrome in women. Women with this medical problem fail to produce a sufficient amount of tears to provide proper lubrication to the eyes. Researchers found that women with the highest intake of omega-3 fatty acids were 17 percent less likely to have dry eye syndrome than women with the lowest intake of these fatty acids. The omega-3 fatty acids in tuna appeared to be particularly beneficial. "These findings are consistent with anecdotal clinical observations and postulated biological mechanisms."[21]

In 2005 *The Journal of Neuroscience* published the results of research on the association between consumption of omega-3 by mice and Alzheimer's disease. Researchers found that when mice ate higher amounts of omega-3, they had significantly lower rates of Alzheimer's disease. People with Alzheimer's have a buildup of plaques of sticky amyloid protein in the brain. Mice with higher levels of omega-3 consumption had 70 percent less buildup of this protein. The researchers believe that omega-3 may well help control the ever escalating rates of Alzheimer's, which now affects about 4.5 million Americans and their families.[22]

An article published in 2002 in the *Journal of the American Medical Association* examined the relationship between intake of omega-3 in women and the incidence of coronary heart disease. Researchers found that the women who consumed more omega-3s had significantly lower rates of coronary heart disease and lower rates of death from heart disease.[23]

On the other hand, after reviewing thousands of scientific papers and abstracts, researchers concluded in a 2006 article in the *British Medical Journal* that omega-3 fats do not have a clear effect on total mortality, combined cardiovascular events, or cancer.[24] Upon adding omega-3 to their diets, some people improved but others became ill. In a July 2007 issue of *Townsend Letter: The Examiner of Alternative Medicine*, famed cardiologist Dean Ornish advises people who have congestive heart failure, chronic recurrent angina (heart pain), or signs that the heart does not receive a sufficient amount of blood, such as pain during exercise, against taking omega-3. Why? Ornish explains that heart blood cells that receive too little blood become "hyper-excitable." Omega-3 calms those cells. "In congestive heart failure, some of the heart tissue has turned into ineffective scar tissue. Consequently, people who already lack blood flow to the heart need even the hyper-excitable cells to pump blood."[25] Ornish believes, however, that most people benefit from consumption of omega-3s.

There is now some good evidence that children with attention-deficit/hyperactivity disorder (ADHD) may be helped by omega-3 (and omega-6) supplementation. An Australian study published in 2007 in the *Journal of Developmental and Behavioral Pediatrics* divided a group of children with ADHD, between the ages of seven and twelve, into three groups. One group took the omega-3/omega-6 supplement; a second group took the supplement and a multivitamin; the third group took placebos. An article published on April 17, 2007, in *PR Newswire Europe* summarized the findings. "Results released from the largest, clinical-based omega-3 and omega-6 trial of its kind show that supplementation with fatty acids relieves the symptoms of ADHD, adding to a growing body of evidence that nutritional intervention can directly benefit children who have issues with inattention, hyperactivity and impulsivity."[26]

MONOUNSATURATED FATS

Monounsaturated fats, such as olive oil, canola oil, and peanut oil, have long been recognized as excellent for heart health. An 2007 article in *Food & Fitness Advisor* notes that, "Monounsaturated fat is the best for heart health, because it decreases the LDL, or 'bad' cholesterol as well as total cholesterol but increases the HDL, or 'good' cholesterol."[27]

Probably the best known monounsaturated fat is olive oil, the fat that is part of the Mediterranean diet. The positive role that the Mediterranean diet may play in cardiovascular health has been well documented by many studies. For instance, research presented before the spring 2007 annual meeting of the American College of Cardiology described a study of 202 individuals who had suffered a heart attack within the previous six weeks. Fifty of these subjects were placed on the American Heart Association low-fat diet, which required an intake of no more than 30 percent fat; fifty-one were placed on the Mediterranean diet, which allowed an intake of 40 percent fat. One hundred were not placed on any special diet. "After four years, 83 percent of those on the low-fat or Mediterranean diets hadn't suffered another heart attack, stroke, or other heart problems, compared to only 53 percent of the others."[28]

In recent years, researchers have determined that olive oil has the potential to do more than protect cardiovascular disease. For example, a 2006 article published in *Archives of Neurology* examined the association between the Mediterranean diet and Alzheimer's disease. Researchers found that people who adhere to the Mediterranean diet have a reduced risk for developing Alzheimer's disease.[29] In fact, people who followed the diet quite strictly "had a 68 percent lower risk of Alzheimer's compared with those who had the lowest adherence."[30]

In 2007 the *Journal of Agricultural and Food Chemistry* reported on a laboratory study that examined the role that olive oil may play in the prevention of peptic ulcers and some gastric cancers caused by *Helicobacter pylori* bacterium. Apparently, olive oil contains abundant amounts of polyphenols, powerful antioxidants that help make fruits and vegetables so healthful. Researchers found that, in the stomach, the polyphenols exerted a strong antibacterial activity. "These results open the possibility of considering virgin olive oil a chemopreventive agent for peptic ulcer or gastric cancer."[31]

A 2005 article in *Nature* notes that newly pressed extra-virgin olive oil contains oleocanthal, a compound that acts "as a natural anti-inflammatory compound that has a potency and profile similar to that of ibuprofen."[32] Still another study, published in 2006 in *Current*

Pharmaceutical Biotechnology, notes that researchers found that oleic acid, the primary monounsaturated fat in olive oil, may "suppress the overexpression and HER2 (erbB-2), a well-characterized oncogene playing a key role in the etiology, invasive progression and metastasis in several human cancers."[33]

Be aware that heating olive oil breaks down some of its antioxidants. But unless a cook heats the oil until it begins to smoke, it should retain most of the benefits. Nuts are another source of monounsaturated fats. A study published in a 2007 issue of *Lipids* added four weeks of forty to ninety grams per day consumption of macadamia nuts to the diets of seventeen men with high levels of blood cholesterol. Researchers found that the consumption of the nuts "modifies favorably the biomarkers of oxidative stress, thrombosis, and inflammation, the risk factors for coronary artery disease, despite the increase in dietary fat intake."[34] The researchers conclude that macadamia nuts may well play a role in preventing coronary artery disease. Almonds are also a wonderful source of monounsaturated fat. For those worried about weight gain from consuming nuts, which are high in fat content, there is an interesting study published in 2007 in *British Journal of Nutrition.* Researchers found that even after eating a daily 344-calorie serving of almonds for ten weeks, there was no change in body weight. The subjects simply ate smaller amounts of other foods.[35]

BAD FATS

There are a few fats that are known to be unhealthful. These include saturated fats, which are most often found in animal products such as whole milk and red meat. At room temperature, saturated fats are solid or waxy. Coconut oil, palm oil, and other tropical oils are also high in saturated fat.

Trans fats, which are also known as trans fatty acids, are formed when hydrogen is added to vegetable oil, a process known as hydrogenation. This makes the fat harder and less likely to spoil. Many foods contain trans fats, including commercial bakery products, shortenings, and some margarines. The human body does not make trans fats and does not need them. It is of interest that a number of cities throughout the United States are prohibiting their use in restaurants. A 2007 issue of the *Harvard Health Letter* notes that trans fats are "now seen as the really bad fat. Beyond its effect on cholesterol, trans fat seems to make platelets 'stickier' (making blood clots more likely), stir up inflammation, and promote the production of extra-small LDL particles that are especially damaging to arteries."[36] However, it is important to realize that food labels may indicate that products contain "zero trans fats" when they actually contain no more than one-half gram of trans fat per serving.[37]

A number of studies have shown a direct association between intake of bad fats and increased risk for certain medical problems. Thus, an article published in 2007 in *Cancer Causes & Control* reported that there is "some evidence" that the consumption of beef, lamb, eggs, dairy, fat, or cholesterol "may increase the risk of pancreatic cancer."[38] Another study, published in the *American Journal of Clinical Nutrition* in 2008, determined that people who frequently eat saturated and trans fats have increased rates of subclinical atherosclerosis.[39] And still another study published in 2007 in *Circulation* concluded that after covariates were adjusted, "high trans fat consumption remains a significant risk factor for coronary heart disease."[40] Those with the highest levels of trans fatty acids in their blood had three times the risk of developing coronary heart disease as those with the lowest levels.[41]

For women having trouble conceiving, a 2007 study published in the *American Journal of Clinical Nutrition* has important information. Using data from the Nurses' Health Study, Harvard Medical School researchers found that even small amounts of trans fats have the potential to cause increases in infertility. Hence, a woman who consumes 2,000 calories per day and who obtains only 2 percent of her calories from trans fats, eats about four grams per day of trans fat or about the amount of trans fats in one doughnut. So, very small amounts of trans fats are able to have a dramatic effect on fertility. "Obtaining two percent of energy from trans fats rather than from monounsaturated fats was associated with a more than doubled risk of ovulatory infertility."[42]

CONCLUSIONS

In the past, all fats were usually clumped together and considered bad for one's health. More recently, it has become quite evident that while some fats are indeed unhealthful and should play a very limited role in the diet, there are fats that should be part of the daily diet. Just about everyone would benefit from more monounsaturated fats, and most people should be adding increased amounts of foods with omega-3s. On the other hand, trans fats should be avoided and saturated fats should be avoided or seriously limited.

TOPICS FOR DISCUSSION

1. Describe your typical breakfast, lunch, and dinner and what type of fats you are eating.

2. Now, analyze the fats you are eating. Are you eating sufficient amounts of the good fats and low amounts of the bad fats?

3. If you are eating too many bad fats and too few good fats, discuss the ways that you can make modifications in your diet.

4. List your five favorite foods that are high in fat. Think of ways to make them healthier.

5. Discuss ways to improve the fat-portion of the diet followed by your entire family. For example, instead of using butter when you cook vegetables, add a little olive oil.

NOTES

1. Rosemary Stanton, *Good Fats Bad Fats* (New York: Marlowe & Company, 2002), 10.

2. Rosemary Stanton, *Good Fats Bad Fats*, 11.

3. Cynthia Sass, "Oil Is Well!" *Prevention* (December 2007) 59: 75.

4. Hannah Wallace, "The New Good Fat: Omega-3s: Good. Omega-6s: Bad. Except for CLA, a Member of the Omega-6 Family that May Help Fight Weight Gain, Allergies, and More. *Natural Health* (July—August 2007) 37: 89–92.

5. Hannah Wallace, "The New Good Fat: Omega-3s.

6. Hannah Wallace, "The New Good Fat: Omega-3s.

7. Linda Antinoro, "Omega-3-Fortified Foods: Fish Out of Water or Healthful Solution to Diet?" *Environmental Nutrition* (July 2007) 30: 1.

8. Nancy Duncan, "Might Omegas," *Women's Health* (December 2006) 3: 47.

9. Cory SerVaas, "How Do You Do the Omega Balance?" *Saturday Evening Post* (July—August 2005) 277: 99.

10. Janice K. Kiecolt-Glaser, Martha A. Belury, Kyle Porter, David Q. Beversdorf, Stanley Lemeshow, and Ronald Glaser, "Depressive Symptoms. Omega-6: Omega-3 Fatty Acids, and Inflammation in Older Adults," *Psychosomatic Medicine* (April 2007) 69: 217–24.

11. "Omega-3 Fatty Acid Levels as a Predictor of Future Suicide Risk," *Brown University Psychopharmacology Update* (September 2006) 17: 1–4.

12. Joseph Hibbeln, Levi R. G. Nieminen, and William E. M. Lands, "Increasing Homicide Rates and Linoleic Acid Consumption Among Five Western Countries, 1961–2000," *Lipids* (December 2004) 39: 1207–13.

13. Millie Hughes-Fulford, Raymond R. Tjandrawinata, Chai-Fei Li, and Sina Sayyah, "Arachidonic Acid, An Omega-6 Fatty Acid, Induces Cytoplasmic Phospholipase A2 in Prostate Carcinoma Cells," *Carcinogenesis* (September 2005) 26: 1520–1526.

14. "Omega-6 Link to Prostate Cancer," *GP* (August 12, 2005) 2.

15. "Excess Dietary Omega-6 Speeds Breast Cancer by Altering Gene Activity," *Women's Health Weekly* (November 11, 2004) 4.

16. Evelyn Tribole, *The Ultimate Omega-3 Diet* (New York: McGraw-Hill, 2007) 182.

17. Evelyn Tribole, *The Ultimate Omega-3 Diet*, 186–187.

18. Hirotsugu Ueshima, Jeremiah Stamler, Paul Elliott, Queenie Chan, et al., "Food Omega-3 Fatty Acid Intake of Individuals (Total, Linolenic Acid, Long-Chain) and Their Blood Pressure," *Hypertension* (August 1, 2007) 50: 313–19.

19. "New Study Shows Fish Oil Supplementation Benefits Arthritic Patients," *Townsend Letter for Doctors and Patients* (October 2005) 267: 16.

20. "New Study Shows Fish Oil Supplementation Benefits Arthritic Patients," 16.

21. Biljana Miljanovic, Komal A. Trivedi, M. Reza Dana, Jaffrey P. Gilbard, Julie E. Buring, and Debra A. Schaumberg, "Relation Between Dietary N-3 and N-6 Fatty Acids and Clinically Diagnosed Dry Eye Syndrome in Women," *The American Journal of Clinical Nutrition* (October 2005) 82: 887–93.

22. Giselle P. Lim, Frédéric Calon, Takashi Morihara, Fusheng Yang, et al., "A Diet Enriched with the Omega-3 Fatty Acid Docosahexaenoic Acid Reduces Amyloid Burden in an Aged Alzheimer Mouse Model," *The Journal of Neuroscience* (March 23, 2005) 25: 3032–40.

23. Frank B. Hu, Leslie Bronner, Walter C. Willett, Meir J. Stampfer, et al., "Fish and Omega-3 Fatty Acid Intake and Risk of Coronary Heart Disease in Women," *Journal of the American Medical Association* (April 10, 2002) 287: 1815–21.

24. Lee Hooper, Rachel L. Thompson, Roger A. Harrison, Carolyn D. Summerbell, et al., "Risks and Benefits of Omega-3 Fats for Mortality, Cardiovascular Disease, and Cancer: Systematic Review," *British Medical Journal* (April 1, 2006) 332: 752–60.

25. Julie Klotter, "Omega-3 Warning," *Townsend Letter: The Examiner of Alternative Medicine* (July 2007) 288: 46–47.

26. "New Published Trial Bolsters Evidence that Omega-3 Fish Can Benefit Children with ADHD Symptoms," *PR Newswire Europe* (April 17, 2007).

27. "Cooking Oil Comparison: What's Healthiest for Your Heart? Olive, Canola, and Peanut Oils Get the Highest Marks in Terms of Healthy Fats, Versatility, and Flavor," *Food & Fitness Advisor* (July 2007) 10: 8–9.

28. "'Healthy' Fats Just as Beneficial as Low-Fat Diet," *Heart Advisor* (June 2007) 10: 2.

29. Scarmeas, Nikolaos, Yaakov Stern, Richard Mayeux, and Jose A. Luchsinger. "Mediterranean Diet, Alzheimer Disease, and Vascular Mediation," *Archives of Neurology* (December 2006) 63: 1709–1717.

30. "Eating a Mediterranean Diet Might Ward Off Alzheimer's," *Focus on Healthy Aging* (January 2007) 10: 2.

31. Concepción Romero, Eduardo Medina, Julio Vargas, Manuel Brenes, and Antonio De Castro, "In Vitro Activity of Olive Oil Polyphenols against *Helicobacter pylori*," *Journal of Agricultural and Food Chemistry* (February 7, 2007) 55: 680–6.

32. Gary K. Beauchamp, Russell S. J. Keast, Diane Morel, Jianming Lin, et al., "Phytochemistry: Ibuprofen-Like Activity in Extra-Virgin Olive Oil," *Nature* (September 1, 2005) 437: 45–46.

33. Javier A. Menendez and Ruth Lupu, "Mediterranean Dietary Traditions for the Molecular Treatment of Human Cancer: Anti-Oncogenic Actions of the Main Olive Oil's Monounsaturated Fatty Acid Oleic Acid," *Current Pharmaceutical Biotechnology* (December 2006) 7: 495–502.

34. Manohar L. Garg, Robert J. Blake, Ron B. H. Wills, and Edward H. Clayton, "Macadamia Nut Consumption Modulates Favorably Risk Factors for Coronary Artery Disease in Hypercholesterolemic Subjects," *Lipids* (June 2007) 42: 583–7.

35. James Hollis and Richard Mattes, "Effect of Chronic Consumption of Almonds on Body Weight in Healthy Humans," *British Journal of Nutrition* (September 2007) 98: 651–6.

36. "Time to Fatten Up Our Diets," *Harvard Health Letter* (September 2007).

37. "When Zero Isn't Nothing," *Harvard Review of Health News* (August 21, 2007).

38. June M. Chan, Furong Wang, and Elizabeth A. Holly, "Pancreatic Cancer, Animal Protein and Dietary Fat in a Population-Based Study," *Cancer Causes & Control* (December 2007) 18: 1153–67.

39. Anwar T. Merchant, Linda E. Kelemen, Lawrence de Koning, Eva Lonn, et al., "Interrelation of Saturated Fat, Trans Fat, Alcohol Intake, and Subclinical Atherosclerosis," *American Journal of Clinical Nutrition* (January 2008) 87: 168.

40. Qi Sun, Jing Ma, Hannia Campos, Susan E. Hankinson, et al., "A Prospective Study of Trans Fatty Acids in Erythrocytes and Risk of Coronary Heart Disease," *Circulation* (April 10, 2007) 115: 1858–65.

41. Qi Sun, Jing Ma, et al., "A Prospective Study of Trans Fatty Acids...."

42. Jorge E. Chavarro, Janet W. Rich-Edwards, Bernard A. Rosner, and Walter Willett, *American Journal of Clinical Nutrition* (January 2007) 85: 231–7.

REFERENCES AND RESOURCES

Books

Allport, Susan. *The Queen of Fats.* Berkeley, California: University of California Press, 2006.
Stanton, Rosemary. *Good Fats Bad Fats.* New York: Marlowe & Company, 2002.
Tribole, Evelyn. *The Ultimate Omega-3 Diet.* New York: McGraw-Hill, 2007.

Magazines, Journals, and Newspapers

Antinoro, Linda. "Omega-3-Fortified Foods: Fish Out of Water or Healthful Addition to Diet?" *Environmental Nutrition* (July 2007) 30: 1.
Beauchamp, Gary K., Russell S. J. Keast, Diane Morel, Jianming Lin, et al. "Phytochemistry: Ibuprofen-Like Activity in Extra-Virgin Olive Oil." *Nature* (September 1, 2005) 437: 45–6.
Chan, June M., Furong Wang, and Elizabeth A. Holly. "Pancreatic Cancer, Animal Protein, and Dietary Fat in a Population-Based Study." *Cancer Causes & Control* (December 2007) 18: 1153–67.
Chavarro, Jorge E., Janet W. Rich-Edwards, Bernard A. Rosner, and Walter C. Willett. "Dietary Fatty Acid Intakes and the Risk of Ovulatory Infertility." *American Journal of Clinical Nutrition* (January 2007) 85: 231.
Colbert, Brandy. "Trans Fat Forestalls Fertility." *Vegetarian Times* (May–June 2007) 350: 16.
"Cooking Oil Comparison: What's Healthiest for You Heart? Olive, Canola, and Peanut Oils Get the Highest Marks in Terms of Healthy Fats, Versatility, and Flavor." *Food & Fitness Advisor* (July 2007) 10: 8–9.
Duncan, Nancy. "Mighty Omegas." *Women's Health* (December 2006) 3: 47.
"Excess Dietary Omega-6 Speeds Breast Cancer by Altering Gene Activity." *Women's Health Weekly* (November 11, 2004) 4.
"Eating a Mediterranean Diet Might Ward Off Alzheimer's." *Focus on Healthy Aging* (January 2007) 10: 2.
Garg, Manohar L., Robert J. Blake, Ron B. H. Wills, and Edward H. Clayton. "Macadamia Nut Consumption Modulates Favorably Risk Factors for Coronary Artery Disease in Hypercholesterolemic Subjects." *Lipids* (June 2007) 42: 583–7.

"'Healthy' Fats Just as Beneficial as Low-Fat Diet." *Heart Advisor* (June 2007) 10: 2.

Hibbeln, Joseph, Levi R. G. Nieminen, and William E. M. Lands. "Increasing Homicide Rates and Linoleic Acid Consumption among Five Western Countries, 1961–2000." *Lipids* (December 2004) 39: 1207–13.

Hollis, James and Richard Mattes. "Effects of Chronic Consumption of Almonds on Body Weight in Healthy Humans." *British Journal of Nutrition* (September 2007) 98: 651–6.

Hooper, Lee, Rachel L. Thompson, Roger A. Harrison, Carolyn D. Summerbell, et al. "Risks and Benefits of Omega 3 Fats for Mortality, Cardiovascular Disease, and Cancer: Systematic Review." *British Medical Journal* (April 1, 2006) 332: 752–60.

Hu, Frank B., Leslie Bronner, Walter C. Willett, Meir J. Stampfer, et al. "Fish and Omega-3 Fatty Acid Intake and Risk of Coronary Heart Disease in Women." *Journal of the American Medical Association* (April 10, 2002) 287: 1815–21.

Hughes-Fulford, Millie, Raymond R. Tjandrawinata, Chai-Fei Li, and Sina Sayyah. "Arachidonic Acid, An Omega-6 Fatty Acid, Induces Cytoplasmic Phospholipase A2 in Prostate Carcinoma Cells." *Carcinogenesis* (September 2005) 26: 1520–6.

Kiecolt-Glaser, Janice K., Martha A. Belury, Kyle Porter, David Q. Beversdorf, Stanley Lemeshow, and Ronald Glaser. "Depressive Symptoms, Omega-6: Omega-3 Fatty Acids, and Inflammation in Older Adults." *Psychosomatic Medicine* (April 2007) 69: 217–24.

Klotter, Julie. "Omega-3 Warning." *Townsend Letter: The Examiner of Alternative Medicine* (July 2007) 288: 46–7.

Lim, Giselle P., Frédéric Calon, Takashi Morihara, Fusheng Yang, et al. "A Diet Enriched with the Omega-3 Fatty Acid Docosahexaenoic Acid Reduces Amyloid Burden in Aged Alzheimer Mouse Model." *The Journal of Neuroscience* (March 23, 2005) 25: 3032–40.

Machowetz, Anja, Henrik E. Poulsen, Sindy Gruendel, Allan Weimann, et al. "Effects of Olive Oils on Biomarkers of Oxidative DNA Stress in Northern and Southern Europeans." *The FASEB Journal* (January 2007) 21: 45–52.

Menendez, Javier A. and Ruth Lupu. "Mediterranean Dietary Traditions for the Molecular Treatment of Human Cancer: Anti-Oncogenic Actions of the Main Olive Oil's Monounsaturated Fatty Acid Oleic Acid." *Current Pharmaceutical Biotechnology* (December 2006) 7: 495–502.

Merchant, Anwar T., Linda E. Kelemen, Lawrence de Koning, Eva Lonn, et al. "Interrelation of Saturated Fat, Trans Fat, Alcohol Intake, and Subclinical Atherosclerosis." *American Journal of Clinical Nutrition* (January 2008) 87: 168.

Mihm, Stephen. "Does Eating Salmon Lower the Murder Rate?" *The New York Times Magazine* (April 16, 2006), 18.

Miljanovic, Biljana, Komal A. Trivedi, M. Reza Dana, Jeffrey P. Gilbard, Julie E. Buring, and Debra A. Schaumberg. "Relation Between Dietary N-3 and N-6 Fatty Acids and Clinically Diagnosed Dry Eye Syndrome in Women." *The American Journal of Clinical Nutrition* (October 2005) 82: 887–93.

"New Published Trial Bolsters Evidence that Omega-3 Fish Oil Can Benefit Children with ADHD Symptoms." *PR Newswire Europe* (April 17, 2007) NA.

"New Study Shows Fish Oil Supplementation Benefits Arthritis Patients." *Townsend Letter for Doctors and Patients* (October 2005) 267: 16.

"Omega-6 Link to Prostate Cancer." *GP* (August 12, 2005), 2.

"Omega-6 Fatty Acids Linked to Depression and Inflammation." *Food & Fitness Advisor* (July 2007) 10: 2.

"Omega-3 Fatty Acid Levels as a Predictor of Future Suicide Risk." *Brown University Psychopharmacology Update* (September 2006) 17: 1–4.

Romero, Concepción, Edwardo Medina, Julio Vargas, Manuel Brenes, and Antonio De Castro. "In Vitro Activity of Olive Oil Polyphenols Against *Helicobacter pylori.*" *Journal of Agricultural and Food Chemistry* (February 7, 2007) 55: 680–6.

Sass, Cynthia. "Oil Is Well!" *Prevention* (December 2007) 59: 75.

Scarmeas, Nikolaos, Yaakov Stern, Richard Mayeux, and Jose A. Luchsinger. "Mediterranean Diet, Alzheimer Disease, and Vascular Mediation." *Archives of Neurology* (December 2006) 63: 1709–17.

SerVaas, Cory. "How Do You Do the Omega Balance?" *Saturday Evening Post* (July—August 2005) 277: 99.

Sinn, Natalie and Janet Bryan. "Effect of Supplementation with Polyunsaturated Fatty Acids and Micronutrients on Learning and Behavior Problems Associated with Child ADHD." *Journal of Developmental & Behavioral Pediatrics* (August 2007) 28: 82–91.

Sun, Qi, Jing Ma, Hannia Campos, Susan E. Hankinson, et al. "A Prospective Study of Trans Fatty Acids in Erythrocytes and Risk of Coronary Heart Disease." *Circulation* (April 10, 2007) 115: 1858–65.

"Time to Fatten Up Our Diets." *Harvard Health Letter* (September 2007) NA.

Ueshima, Hirotsugu, Jeremiah Stamler, Paul Elliott, Queenie Chan, et al. "Food Omega-3 Fatty Acid Intake of Individuals (Total, Linolenic Acid, Long-Chain) and Their Blood Pressure." *Hypertension* (August 2, 2007) 50: 313–19.

Wallace, Hannah. "The New Good Fat: Omega-3s. Omega-6s: Bad. Except for CLA, a Member of the Omega-6 Family that May Help Fight Weight Gain, Allergies, and More." *Natural Health* (July—August 2007) 37: 89–92.

"When Zero Isn't Nothing." *Harvard Reviews of Health News* (August 21, 2007) NA.

Yost, Debora. "Powerful Protection Against Heart Disease, Cancer, and Inflammation." *Life Extension* (September 2007).

Websites

American Dietetic Association
www.eatright.org

U. S. Food and Drug Administration
http://www.fda.gov

Harvard School of Public Health
http://www.hsph.harvard.edu

Chapter 5

Wild versus Farm-Raised Fish

Not that long ago, the average American ate very little fish. A typical dinner was more likely some form of meat, vegetable, and carbohydrate, such as a hamburger, peas, and mashed potatoes. When fish was included in a meal, it often came from the freezer section of the supermarket and was breaded—the ever so common fish sticks.

Today, fresh fish is ubiquitous. It is almost impossible to imagine a supermarket without a sizeable department devoted entirely to fresh fish. Stores that sell fresh fish may be found even in smaller towns throughout the country. Clearly, more and more Americans are making fish a regular part of their diets.

According to an article published in 2007 in *Feedstuffs*, in 2006 Americas ate an average of 16.5 pounds of fish and shellfish. That is a 2 percent increase over the 2005 consumption figure of 16.2 pounds. In 2006 Americans consumed almost five billion pounds of seafood. About 83 percent of this fish is imported. So it should not surprise anyone that only the Chinese and Japanese consume more fish than Americans.[1]

BENEFITS OF EATING FISH

The Better Health Channel notes that there are a number of benefits to eating fish. It is high in protein and is "an excellent source of omega 3 fatty acids." The consumption of fish has the potential to reduce the risk of various diseases and disorders. Fish is probably best known for lowering the risk for cardiovascular diseases, such as heart disease and stroke. That is because fish increases the elasticity of blood vessels, raises "good" cholesterol, and reduces blood pressure, the risk for blood clots, and inflammation. People with diabetes who eat fish may have better management of their blood sugar levels. The consumption of fish has also been associated with relief from the symptoms of autoimmune

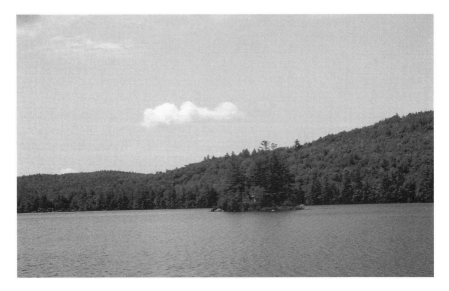

You need not worry about fish treated with antibiotics from this lake in Maine. (Courtesy of Mark A. Goldstein)

disease, psoriasis, and rheumatoid arthritis. And it is believed that children who eat fish are less likely to develop asthma.[2]

Obviously, there is a huge worldwide demand for fish, and this demand can no longer be met by the catching of wild fish. Many of the world's wild fisheries have been overharvested, and, as a result, the amount of fish that may now be obtained has declined considerably.

To fill the gap, the world relies upon fish farming or aquaculture. It has been estimated that about 40 percent of the world's seafood comes from fish farming.[3] Some say that figure is much higher—closer to 50 percent.[4] Because fish obtained via farming tends to be less expensive than wild fish, it makes fresh fish more affordable and available to those with more modest resources. Still, there are people who simply refuse to eat farm-raised fish. The entire wild fish versus aquaculture debate has become enormously controversial.

People are often surprised to learn that fish farming is not a new concept. In fact, there were small fish farms in the ancient civilizations of China, Egypt, and Japan. During the first half of the twentieth century, state and federal researchers developed fish farming methods. By the mid-twentieth century, there were tilapia, shrimp, and catfish farms in the United States. Since then, the industry has exploded in growth. According to the National Aquaculture Association, "aquaculture is the fastest growing sector of US agriculture." Of all types of fish farmed in the United States, the largest in total production is catfish farming. It exceeds 500 million pounds per year. After catfish, there are "(listed according to pounds raised) oysters, trout, crawfish, salmon, clams, tilapia, striped bass, baitfish, and ornamental fishes."[5] But aquaculture is not confined to the United States. It is a huge worldwide industry. "Aquaculture has been one of the fastest growing components of global food production in recent decades, increasing by more than 10 percent a year."[6] This explosion of aquaculture is known as the "Blue Revolution."[7]

But what exactly is aquaculture? How is it defined? According to the Department of Marine Resources of the State of Maine, the common definition of aquaculture "is the farming of aquatic organisms such as fish, shellfish and even plants. The term aquaculture refers to the cultivation of both marine and freshwater species and can range from land-based to open-ocean production."[8] But the site also notes a legal definition for aquaculture. "The culture or husbandry of marine organisms by any person. Storage or any other form of impounding or holding of wild marine organisms, without more, shall not qualify as aquaculture. In order to quality as aquaculture a project must involve affirmative action by the lessee to improve the growth rate or quality of the marine organism."[9]

In a practical sense, how does fish farming work? Of course, fish farming varies from farm to farm. To provide an example, take the case of Wild West Steelhead in Saskatchewan, Canada, which breeds steelhead trout, a type of rainbow trout. The fish begin as fertilized eggs that are hatched in the company's hatchery. When the fish are three months old, they are transferred to growing pens in Lake Diefenbaker.

For the next eighteen to twenty-four months the fish grow in the pens. When they are around two kilograms in size, they are harvested. Every year, the business processes about 600,000 fish. No antibiotics are used. Because the pens need to be periodically inspected, several employees are certified scuba divers.[10]

NEGATIVE ASPECTS OF FISH FARMING

So why is fish farming so controversial? Not all fish farms are like the Wild West Steelhead. A 2007 article in *Natural Life* states that "fish farming can pollute river and streams, while harming wild fish. Plus, feeding farmed fish can be problematic, intensifying pressure on the ocean stocks."[11] Moreover, all too often, in an attempt to raise more fish, they are grown in crowded and confined areas, which increase levels of stress and opportunities to pass along various diseases. (The David Suzuki Foundation notes that as many 50,000 salmon may be kept in one net-cage.[12]) Outside the United States, it is not uncommon for these diseases to be treated with medications, such as antibiotics. To help prevent disease, disinfectants and pesticides may be used. In 2005 the FDA rejected close to 3,000 seafood shipments because they contained antibiotic residues. (Because only 1–2 percent of all imported seafood is tested, the exact amount of treated fish that enters the United States is unknown.)[13]

There also is concern about pollutants in farmed fish, especially from fish that has been imported. Often the fish is obtained from smaller farmers, which may or may not be following the few existing regulations. Barry Cost-Pierce, the director of the Rhode Island Sea Grant College Program and professor of Fisheries & Aquaculture at the University of Rhode Island noted, "We're letting tainted products come into the United States with improper testing. Everybody in the scientific community knows about these issues, but there's no government hammer behind them."[14]

Concentrations of PCBs

Early in 2004, the results of an important study were published in *Science*. A team of researchers, led by Ronald Hites of Indiana University, measured contaminants in about 700 farmed and wild salmon from different locations throughout the world. They found that the concentrations of polychlorinated biphenyls (PCBs) and other contaminants were consistently higher in farmed salmon, but at limits well below those set by the federal government. Farm salmon had more than seven times the concentrations of PCBs than wild salmon. Furthermore, the concentrations were higher in salmon from European locations than salmon from North or South American locations. Most likely, the farmed salmon obtained these contaminants from their food, which consisted of fish meal and oil from fish with higher levels of contaminants. Because of their findings, the researchers suggested that most consumers should limit their intake of farmed salmon to no more than one meal per month. Wild salmon may be consumed up to eight times per month. The researchers noted, "Risk analysis indicates that consumption of farmed Atlantic salmon may pose health risks that detract from the beneficial effects of fish consumption."[15]

A 2004 article in *The New York Times* that reported on the study's findings noted that Terry Troxell, of the Food and Drug Administration, said that there was no reason for unease. In the article, Troxell is quoted as follows: "We certainly don't think there's a public health concern here. Our advice to consumers is not to alter their consumption of farmed or wild salmon." Troxell noted that most of the contaminants were found in the skin and the fat just under the skin. "Most people aren't eating the skin. And when salmon is cooked, you lose a considerable amount of fat, and so the levels go down quite a bit."[16]

In another article in the same issue of *Science*, Charles Santerre, a toxicologist at Purdue University who is also a consultant with the industry group Salmon of the Americas, contends that people who avoid farmed salmon lose the nutritional benefits that it offers. He also underscored that the contaminants levels in farmed salmon are well below what the federal government permits. According to Santerre, "In my view, the study says we should be eating more farmed salmon."[17]

A week later, *The New York Times* ran an editorial that addressed the farm versus wild salmon question. It noted that the once per month suggestion was against the advice usually offered about fish. Most often, the editorial said, heart experts recommend people eat at least two fish meals per week. Fatty fish, such as salmon, tuna, or mackerel, are considered particularly valuable. "The real message of this study is that the fish farming industry needs to clean up its feeding materials to reduce the level of contaminants. It would also be desirable for salmon to be labeled clearly to show whether it was farmed or wild, and where it came from."[18]

A study published in 2005 in *The Journal of Nutrition* evaluated the benefits and risks of consuming farmed and wild salmon. Specifically, it compared the risks of exposure to organic contaminants in salmon to the benefits obtained from consuming salmon's fatty acids. The researchers concluded that the "risk of exposure to contaminants in farmed and wild salmon is partially offset by the fatty acid-associated health benefits."[19] Still, the researchers advise children, women of childbearing age, and women who are pregnant or nursing to minimize their exposure to contaminants and eat wild salmon or other nonfarmed salmon sources of fatty acids. Charles Santerre also disagrees with that statement. "I think it is unconscionable to direct pregnant women away from farmed salmon."[20] Santerre believes that the omega-3 fatty acids are needed for brain development, and they increase a child's cognitive development and may reduce the risk of preterm births.

Infecting Other Fish

Canadian researchers have raised another potentially disturbing side to fish farming. In a December 14, 2007, article in *Science,* Martin Krkosek, a fisheries ecologist at the University of Alberta, and other researchers noted that as juvenile wild salmon travel in rivers and streams, they may become infected with parasites from nearby fish farms. "We show that recurrent louse infections of wild juvenile pink salmon (Oncorhynchus gorbuscha), all associated with salmon farms, have depressed wild pink salmon populations and placed them on a trajectory toward rapid local extinction. The louse-induced mortality of pink salmon is commonly over 89% and exceeds previous fishing mortality. If outbreaks continue, then local extinction is certain, and a 99% collapse in pink salmon population abundance is expected in four salmon generations."[21]

A December 14, 2007, article in *The New York Times* contained comments on the researchers' findings. Fisheries biologist from the University of Washington, Ray Hilborn, said that, "the high-density fish farms are natural breeding grounds for pathogens." At the same time, Hilborn said that pink salmon are smaller than sockeye or chinook, which may make them more vulnerable to sea lice. Hilborn also said that the study pointed out "serious concerns about proposed aquaculture for other species, such as cod, halibut, and sablefish."[22] Meanwhile, Fisheries and Oceans Canada, the Canadian governmental agency in charge of overseeing aquaculture while protecting wild fish, noted that there was no direct cause and effect relationship established between the sea lice and salmon mortality.[23] Brian Riddell, an agency ecologist, said that it is important to consider other factors, such as fishing practices, climate change, and logging. It is wrong "to become overly focused on a single point."[24]

Printed on the same day, an article in the *Washington Post* offered additional observations on the study. Andrew Rosenberg, a former deputy director of the National Oceanic and Atmospheric Administration (NOAA) said, "We're not talking about being mean to some individual fish; we're talking about a possible extinction within the next few years" of pink salmon.[25] On the other hand, Kevin Amos, aquatic coordinator for NOAA's Marine Fisheries Service said that a number of factors affect salmon runs. "We have to consider all things when establishing a cause and effect in aquaculture, and in this case the authors did not do that."[26]

Salmon Escaping from Pens

Then, there is the problem of the salmon that escape from their pens. A 2005 article in *The Chronicle of Higher Education* notes that every year "millions of salmon escape from pens around the world." In addition to competing with the native fish for resources, "they often interbreed with wild fish and reduce the strength of threatened populations."[27] Rebecca J. Goldburg, a senior scientist at Environmental Defense, an environmental organization in New York, said that the resulting hybrid is not prepared to live in the wild.[28] A 2003 National Geographic News article notes that, "hybrid fish have poor survival rates at sea and are unable to find their way back to freshwater to spawn."[29] Farmed fish are bred to grow quickly not to hunt at sea, jump waterfalls, and locate a specific river. The article estimates that two million farm salmon escape from their marine cages in the North Atlantic each year. That is "equivalent to about 50 percent of all wild adult salmon in the sea.... Research suggests as many as one-third of adult salmon entering Norwegian rivers are farmed fish, while it's estimated they now outnumber native salmon by ten to one in some North American rivers."[30]

One possible solution to this problem is to locate the pens a mile or more offshore in 100 feet of water, instead of the usual use of bays or channels. Because pens are closed at the top, it is far more difficult to escape. Besides, water currents wash away pollution and disease organisms. People who cherish using the coastline for recreational purposes are less likely to complain. Still, such offshore pens could be hit by hurricanes, and there is always the problem of ocean predators and the costs associated with transporting the crew and equipment.

SOME FISH CLEANSE THE WATER

But, amazingly, there are some types of fish—bivalve shellfish such as oysters, clams, and mussels—that actually make water cleaner. They filter seawater and feed on plankton and floating particles in the water. According to Hauke Kite-Powell, a researcher at the Woods Hole Oceanographic Institution, "Shellfish are by far the most cost-effective strategy to control pollution. It's about maximizing all the variables to come up with a good policy."[31] So, fish farmers are beginning to grow these bivalve shellfish near their regular fish farms, a process known as polyculture. Seaweeds serve a similar function. Goldburg contends that this form of fish farming is far better for the environment. "Recycling nutrients is a foundation of sustainable agriculture. You get another crop, and you cut pollution."[32] These types of fish farms are now located in countries as diverse as Australia, China, Chile, Canada, Israel, South Africa, and Thailand.[33] An article published in 2007 in *Environment* emphasizes the need "to progress from the limited perspective of ultimately unsustainable fish and shrimp monocultures to a balanced ecosystem approach that respects the environment and includes seaweeds and shellfish as health and valuable products of each fish and shrimp farm."[34] That would require a change in the current fish eating paradigm. "Consumers would have to eat more marine plants and shellfish and fewer of the popular, large carnivorous fish and shrimp that generate aquaculture's worst environmental impacts."[35]

Even the most diehard fish fan must find reading this chapter unsettling. If the figures are correct and millions of fish are escaping from their pens and breeding with wild fish, then the distinction between the two becomes blurred. Just because a fish, such as salmon, is swimming in the wild, there is obviously no guarantee that it is wild. Further, what is labeled as "wild" may actually be "farmed." In March 2005 *The New York Times* purchased "wild" salmon at eight New York City stores for as much as $29 per pound. However, when the salmon was tested, it was determined that six of the eight pieces of salmon were "farmed." Apparently, the testers found that one of the samples has originally been farmed before escaping into the wild. Around the same time, *The New York Times* telephoned twenty-five New York City stores to determine the availability of wild salmon. Of these, twenty-three said that they had it in stock. "The findings mirror suspicions of many in the seafood business. That wild salmon could not be so available from November to March, the off-season."[36]

A 2004 article in the *Annals of Internal Medicine* noted that the U.S. Environmental Protection Agency (EPA) has identified PCBs as a probable carcinogen or cancer causing agent. Animal studies have found an association between PCBs and liver and breast cancer, endocrine and neurological problems, and it may even increase the risk of cardiovascular disease. "In children, PCB exposure in utero and from breast milk consumption has been linked with neurodevelopmental delays, impaired cognition, immune problems, and alterations in male reproductive organs."[37]

There is also some evidence that PCBs have an effect on the central nervous system. A study published in 2001 in *Environmental Health Perspectives* compared the intellectual functioning of 101 adults between the ages of forty-nine and eight-six who ate more than twenty-four pounds of sport-caught fish per year from Lake Michigan with seventy-nine people who ate less than six pounds of Lake Michigan fish per year. Researchers found that "PCB exposure during adulthood was associated with impairments in memory and learning.... These results are consistent with previous research showing an association between *in utero* PCB exposure and impairments of memory during infancy and childhood."[38]

So what should the typical consumer do? First, it is important to realize that although fatty fish are considered the best sources for omega-3 fatty acids, there are other foods that contain these fatty acids. These include flaxseed, soybeans, walnuts, and canola. Furthermore, consider some recommendations provided by the Association of Reproductive Health Professionals and the Physicians for Social Responsibility. Because any PCBs are more likely in the fatty sections of a fatty fish, when preparing a fatty fish, such as salmon or bluefish, trim the fattier area—the belly, top of the back, and dark meat along the side. Before cooking, puncture or remove the skin. That enables fat to drain. Do not fry the fish. Instead, steam, roast, grill, or broil it. Discard any fatty drippings. The two organizations recommend that "fatty fish consumption should be limited to one to two meals per month." To compensate for the loss of health benefits derived from eating more fish, people are advised to make "basic lifestyle changes to help ensure cardiovascular health."[39] As for children, "to reduce the risk of high exposure to pollutants from over-consumption of any one fish, parents should be advised to teach children from an early age to enjoy a variety of ... low-PCB fish and shellfish."[40]

Despite all the problems, an article published at the end of 2007 in *Global Agenda* calls for an increase in fish farming to meet the increasing food demands of growing populations. Moreover, the article offered some solutions to the problems associated with fish farming. Instead of raising so many carnivorous fish, like salmon, raise more vegetarian fish, such as tilapia and catfish. Move fish pens to better locations and away from wild salmon runs. Another idea is to design self-contained ponds that avoid the dumping of feces and uneaten food onto the marine floor. The article ends with an optimistic thought. "Compared to terrestrial agriculture, fish farming is young, and it has a lot of growing up to do. Like farming, it causes environmental problems but offers great benefits. The world will have to find solutions to the first in order properly to enjoy the second."[41]

CONCLUSION

By reviewing this chapter it becomes evident that the there is often not a clear distinction between wild and farm-raised fish, and there are problems with both types of fish. Wild fisheries have been overfished, and a fish described as "wild" may or may not actually be wild. It may well have contaminants, and, in all probability, it will be expensive. Farmed fish, while less costly than wild fish, may have been grown in terrible conditions and exposed to a host of different agents and contaminants. Perhaps with increased awareness of these issues, there will be more impetus for corrective action.

TOPICS FOR DISCUSSION

1. How did you feel about eating fish before you read this chapter? How do you feel about eating fish now?

2. Has reading this chapter motivated you to learn more about wild and farmed fish? Why or why not?

3. Are you concerned about the levels of contaminants in the fish you eat? Why or why not?

4. Do you eat imported fish? Do you believe it is safe? Why or why not?

5. Do you think more imported fish should be inspected? Why or why not?

NOTES

1. Suzi Fraser Dominy, "Seafood Consumption in the U.S. Up for 2006." *Feedstuffs* (July 30, 2007) 79: 10–11.

2. Better Health Channel website, http:///www.betterhealth.vic.gov.au.

3. Jennifer Weeks, "Fish Farming: Is it Safe for Humans and the Environment?" *CQ Researcher* (July 27, 2007) 17: 625.

4. Graeme O'Neill, "Aquaculture Advances: In the Past Decade, Aquaculture Has Become a $100 Billion Global Industry—The Fastest Growing Food-Production Sector Since the Advent of Intensive Agriculture in the 1950s." *Ecos* (April—May 2007) 136: 22–25.

5. National Aquaculture Association website, http://www.thenaa.org.

6. *Mother Jones* website, http://motherjones.com.

7. Jennifer Weeks, "Fish Farming: Is it Safe for Humans and the Environment?" 627.

8. Department of Marine Resources, State of Maine, website, http://www.state.me.us/dmr/index.htm.

9. Department of Marine Resources, State of Maine, website.

10. "True Fish Story: From Luck Lake to Brooklyn: From the Land of Living Skies to the Big Apple, There's No Taste Like Home." *SaskBusiness* (March—April 2007) S3.

11. "How Green is My Diet?" *Natural Life* (September—October 2007) 7–9.

12. David Suzuki Foundation website, http://www.davidsuzuki.org.

13. Jennifer Weeks, "Fish Farming: Is it Safe for Humans and the Environment?" 630.

14. Jennifer Weeks, "Fish Farming: Is it Safe for Humans and the Environment?" 629.

15. Ronald A. Hites, Jeffrey A. Foran, David O. Carpenter, M. Coreen Hamilton, Barbara A. Knuth, Steven J. Schwager. "Global Assessment of Organic Contaminants in Farmed Salmon." *Science* (January 9, 2004) 303: 226–9.

16. Gina Kolata, "Farmed Salmon Have More Contaminants Than Wild Ones, Study Finds." *The New York Times* (January 9, 2004) A12, col 01.

17. Erik Stokstad, "Salmon Survey Stokes Debate About Farmed Fish." *Science* (January 9, 2004) 303: 154—5.

18. "Farmed Salmon, Pro and Con," *The New York Times* (January 17, 2004) A14, col 01.

19. Foran, Jeffrey, David H. Good, David O. Carpenter, M. Coreen Hamilton, Barbara A. Knuth, and Steven J. Schwager, "Quantitative Analysis of the Benefits and Risks of Consuming Farmed and Wild Salmon." *The Journal of Nutrition* (November 2005) 135: 2639–43.

20. Erik Stokstad, "Salmon Survey Stokes Debate About Farmed Fish," 154–5.

21. Martin Krkosek, Jennifer S. Ford, Alexandra Morton, Subhash Lele, Ransom A. Myers, and Mark A. Lewis, "Declining Wild Salmon Populations in Relation to Parasites from Farm Salmon." *Science* (December 14, 2007) 317: 1772–5.

22. Cornelia Dean, "Lice in Fish Farms Endanger Wild Salmon, Study Says." *The New York Times* (December 14, 2007) 157: A10.

23. Cornelia Dean, "Lice in Fish Farms Endanger Wild Salmon, Study Says," A10.

24. Cornelia Dean, "Live in Fish Farms Endanger Wild Salmon, Study Says," A10.

25. Juliet Eilperin and Marc Kaufman, "Salmon Farming May Doom Wild Populations, Study Says," *Washington Post* (December 14, 2007) A28.

26. Juliet Eilperin and Marc Kaufman, "Salmon Farming May Doom Wild Populations, Study Says," A28.

27. Richard Monastersky, "The Hidden Cost of Farming Fish," *The Chronicle of Higher Education* (April 22, 2005) 51: NA.

28. Richard Monastersky, "The Hidden Cost of Farming Fish," NA.

29. James Owen, "Wild-Farm Salmon Hybrids Not Reaching Spawning Grounds?" (October 28, 2003) National Geographic News website, http://news.nationalgeographic.com.

30. James Owen, "Wild-Farm Salmon Hybrids Not Reaching Spawning Grounds?"

31. Paul D. Thacker, "Oysters and Clams Clean Up Dirty Water." *Environmental Science & Technology* (May 15, 2006) 40: 3131–2.

32. Jennifer Weeks, "Fish Farming: Is it Safe for Humans and the Environment?" 633.

33. Amir Neori, Max Troell, Thierry Chopin, Charles Yarish, Alan Critchley, and Alejandro H. Buschmann, "The Need for a Balanced Ecosystem Approach to Blue Revolution Aquaculture," *Environment* (April 2007) 49: 36–43.

34. Amir Neori, Max Troell, Thierry Chopin, Charles Yarish, Alan Critchley, and Alejandro H. Buschmann, "The Need for a Balanced Ecosystem Approach to Blue Revolution Aquaculture," 36–43.

35. Jennifer Weeks, "Fish Farming: Is it Safe for Humans and the Environment?" 633.

36. Marian Burros, "Stores Say Wild, but Tests Say Farm Bred," *The New York Times* (April 10, 2005) A1.

37. J. F. Wilson, "Balancing the Risks and Benefits of Fish Consumption," *Annals of Internal Medicine* (December 21, 2004) 141: 977–80.

38. Susan L. Schantz, Donna M. Gasior, Elena Polverejan, Robert J. McCaffrey, Anne M. Sweeney, Harold E.B. Humphrey, and Joseph C. Gardiner, "Impairments of Memory and Learning in Older Adults Exposed to Polychlorinated Biphenyls Via Consumption of Great Lakes Fish," *Environmental Health Perspectives* (June 2001) 109: 605–11.

39. Association of Reproductive Health Professionals and Physicians for Social Responsibility, "Fish Consumption to Promote Good Health and Minimize Contaminants," (booklet) ARHP and PSR (2004) 10.

40. Association of Reproductive Health Professional and Physicians for Social Responsibility, "Fish Consumption to Promote Good Health and Minimize Contaminants," 11.

41. "Mind the Gap; Green View; The World Needs More Farmed Fish," *Global Agenda* (December 27, 2007) NA.

REFERENCES AND RESOURCES

Books

Association of Reproductive Health Professionals (APHP) and Physicians for Social Responsibility (PSR). *Fish Consumption to Promote Good Health and Minimize Contaminants* (booklet). ARHP and PSR, 2004.

Kallen, Stuart A., editor. *Is Factory Farming Harming America?* Farmington Hills, Michigan: Greenhaven Press, 2006.

Molyneaux, Paul. *Swimming in Circles.* New York: Thunder's Mouth Press, 2007.

Magazines, Journals, and Newspapers

Burros, Marian. "Stores Say Wild Salmon, But Tests Say Farm Bred." *The New York Times* (April 10, 2005) A1(L).

Dean, Cornelia. "Lice in Fish Farms Endanger Wild Salmon, Study Says." *The New York Times* (December 14, 2007) 157: A10(L).

Dominy, Suzi Fraser. "Seafood Consumption in the U.S. for 2006." *Feedstuffs* (July 30, 2007) 79: 10–11.

Eilperin, Juliet and Marc Kaufman. "Salmon Farming May Doom Wild Populations." *Washington Post* (December 14, 2007) A28.

"Farmed Salmon, Pro and Con." *The New York Times* (January 17, 2004) A14, col 01.

Foran, Jeffrey A., David H. Good, David O. Carpenter, M. Coreen Hamilton, Barbara A. Knuth, and Steven J. Schwager. "Quantitative Analysis of the Benefits and Risks of Consuming Farmed and Wild Salmon." *The Journal of Nutrition* (November 2005) 135: 2639–43.

Hites, Ronald A., Jeffery A. Foran, David O. Carpenter, M. Coreen Hamilton, Barbara A. Knuth, and Steven J. Schwager. "Global Assessment of Organic Contaminants in Farmed Salmon." *Science* (January 9, 2004) 303: 226–9.

"How Green is My Diet?" *Natural Life* (September—October 2007) 7–9.

Kolata, Gina. "Farmed Salmon Have More Contaminants Than Wild Ones, Study Finds." *The New York Times* (January 9, 2004) A12, col 01.

Krkosek, Martin, Jennifer S. Ford, Alexandra Morton, Subhash Lele, Ransom A. Myers, and Mark A Lewis. "Declining Wild Salmon Populations in Relation to Parasites from Farm Salmon." *Science* (December 14, 2007) 318: 1772–5.

"Mind the Gap; Green View; The World Needs More Farmed Fish." *Global Agenda* (December 27, 2007) NA.

Monastersky, Richard. "The Hidden Cost of Farming Fish." *The Chronicle of Higher Education* (April 22, 2005) 51.

Neori, Amir, Max Troell, Thierry Chopin, Charles Yarish, Alan Critchley, and Alejandro H. Buschmann. "The Need for a Balanced Ecosystem Approach to Blue Revolution Aquaculture." *Environment* (April 2007) 49: 36–43.

O'Neill, Graeme. "Aquaculture Advances: In the Past Decade, Aquaculture Has Become a $100 Billion Global Industry—The Fastest Growing Food-Production Sector Since the Advent of Intensive Agriculture in the 1950s." *Ecos* (April—May 2007) 136: 22–5.

Owen, James. "Wild-Farm Salmon Hybrids Not Reaching Spawning Ground?" October 28, 2003, National Geographic News website, http://news.nationalgeographic.com.

Pennybacker, Mindy and P.W. McRandle. "Fish and Tips." *Grist Magazine* (February 24, 2004) NA.

Schantz, Susan L., Donna M. Gasior, Elena Polverejan, Robert J. McCaffrey, Anne M. Sweeney, Harold E.B. Humphrey, and Joseph C. Gardiner. "Impairment of Memory and Learning in Older Adults Exposed to Polychlorinated Biphenyls Via Consumption of Great Lakes Fish." *Environmental Health Perspectives* (June 2001) 109(6): 605–11.

Stokstad, Erik. "Salmon Survey Stokes Debate About Farmed Fish." *Science* (January 9, 2004) 303: 154–5.

Thacker, Paul D. "Oysters and Clams Clean Up Dirty Water." *Environmental Science & Technology* (May 15, 2006) 40: 3131–2.

"True Fish Story: From Lucky Lake to Brooklyn: From the Land of Living Skies to the Big Apple, There's No Taste Like Home." *SaskBusiness* (March—April 2007) 28: S3.

Weeks, Jennifer. "Fish Farming: Is it Safe for Humans and the Environment?" *CQ Researcher* (July 27, 2007) 17: 625–48.

Wilson, J.F. "Balancing the Risks and Benefits of Fish Consumption." *Annals of Internal Medicine* (December 21, 2004) 141: 977–80.

Websites

Better Health Channel
http://www.betterhealth.vic.gov.au

David Suzuki Foundation
http://www.davidsuzuki.org

Department of Marine Resources, State of Maine
http://www.state.me.us/dmr/index.htm

Mother Jones
http://motherjones.com

National Aquaculture Association
http://www.thenaa.org

Pure Salmon Campaign
http://www.puresalmon.org

Woods Hole Oceanographic Institute
http://www.whoi.edu

Chapter 6

Food Labeling

Food labels may be a tremendous assistance for people who carefully monitor what they eat, but some labels may present inaccurate or incomplete information. In the mid-1980s, the role of diet in the development of chronic illness was better understood than before, but there were laws that prevented manufacturers from placing nutritional information on food labels. Everything changed in October 1984 when the Kellogg Company and the National Cancer Institute (NCI) joined together to launch a promotional campaign for All-Bran, a high-fiber breakfast cereal. The cereal package contained an explicit health claim for bran cereals in the diet and offered tips from the NCI to reduce the risk of cancer. Although such labeling was against the law, the U.S. Food and Drug Administration took no regulatory action. Other cereal manufacturers soon began to make similar health claims on their products.

These actions triggered a host of controversies between the scientific community, food manufacturers, and regulators. Were these labels appropriate? Were they valid? Did they assist consumers? Amid all the dissension, consumers did not know whom or what to believe.

Nevertheless, the actions of these cereal manufacturers proved to be a catalyst for change. The federal government acted quickly. In just a few years, the food-labeling landscape changed dramatically. Food labels now contain a great deal of information. Consumers appear to be responding. While results vary, a 2005 article in the *American Journal of Clinical Nutrition* notes that between 60 and 80 percent of food shoppers read a label before purchasing a new food product; between 30 and 40 percent indicate that "the label had influenced their choice."[1] What are consumers looking for? A 2006 article in the *American Journal of Clinical Nutrition* indicates "consumers consider calories (58%) and total fat (56%) first, followed by sodium and saturated fat (both at 45%), sugars (42%), cholesterol (39%), and carbohydrates (34%)."[2]

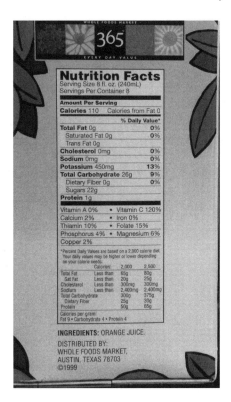

Consumers check food labels to determine calories, sodium, fat, and other ingredients. (Courtesy of Mark A. Goldstein)

Who reads the labels? The International Food Information Council contends that older people, women, and parents are the three groups of people who most often read food labels. "Consumers who are more inclined to read food labels in Canada are those claiming to have very good to excellent eating habits and are knowledgeable about nutrition. U.S. consumers who are interested in health because they have specific health concerns are more likely to look at the NFP [Nutrition Facts panel]."[3] A study published in 2006 in the *Journal of Nutrition Education and Behavior* surveyed 1,139 adults. Of these, 53 percent indicated that they consistently reviewed the Nutrition Facts panels of food products. The most likely to review the panels were "females, those with more educations, and those currently married."[4]

Food labeling is a broad term, and over the years, the federal requirements for food labeling have evolved. Labels now include Nutrition Facts, nutrition-related claims, and an ingredient statement. What are these? The International Food Information Council offers excellent explanations:

Nutrition Facts: This panel, found on the back or side of a package, contains product-specific information about serving size, calories, and nutrients; Percent Daily Value (%DV) based on a 2000 calorie diet; and if the package is large enough, footnotes with Daily Values (DVs) that provides a summary of recommended dietary intakes for important nutrients including dietary fats, sodium, and fiber, among others.

Nutrition-Related Claims: Often located on the front of a food package, these consist of nutrient content claims that describe the amount of a nutrient in the food (e.g. 'low-fat') or health claims, which relate a food or food component to a disease or health-related condition (e.g. 'Calcium may reduce the risk of osteoporosis.').

Ingredient Statement: A list of ingredients found in the food product which are listed in descending order by weight, from the most to the least.[5]

Since the Food Allergen Labeling and Consumer Protection Act (FALCPA) was passed into law and made effective as of January 1, 2006, labels must identify the "potentially allergenic ingredients from any of the eight major allergenic foods: dairy, eggs, fish, shellfish, tree nuts, wheat, peanuts, and soybeans."[6] These allergens account for 90 percent of all food allergies.[7] The warning must be placed near the list of ingredients. (This is not necessary if the major food allergen's common name identifies the food source, e.g., whole wheat flour.) According to the law, a major food allergen is "any ingredient that contains protein derived from any of these eight foods. The plain language declaration [e.g., using the word milk instead of the word casein] requirement of FALCPA also applies to flavorings, coloring, and incidental additives that are or contain a major food allergen."[8] This is of immense importance to the millions of people who suffer from allergies, food intolerances, and illnesses in which certain foods must be avoided, such as celiac disease. And the numbers of affected people just keep rising.

Precautionary allergen statements are also important. For example, although a particular food may not contain an allergen, it may be processed in a plant that also processes that allergen. When that occurs, cross-contamination may take place.

Meanwhile, as of the same date, the Food and Drug Administration (FDA) required that "food manufacturers to list *trans* fat (i.e. trans fatty acids) on Nutrition Facts and some Supplement Facts panels."[9] A 2006 article in the *Mississippi Business Journal* notes that the American Heart Association has indicated that the "consumption of trans fat raises LDL ('bad') cholesterol and lowers HDL ('good') cholesterol, causing the arteries to become clogged and increasing the risk of developing heart disease and stroke."[10] Still, it is important to mention that a label may state that a product has no trans fat when it actually contains 0.5 gram or less per serving.

Food labeling is controlled by several federal government agencies. Most packaged foods, produce, seafood, milk, and eggs are regulated by the Food and Drug Administration, which is part of the U.S.

Department of Health and Human Services. Meat and poultry products are regulated by the Food Safety and Inspection Service (FSIS) in the U.S. Department of Agriculture (USDA). At the same time, the U.S. Federal Trade Commission (FTC) is in charge of food advertising. Throughout the years, a number of acts have formed the basis of food and nutrition labeling. These include the Meat Inspection Act of 1906, the Federal Food, Drug, and Cosmetic Act of 1938, the Poultry Products Inspection Act of 1957, and the Wholesome Meat Act of 1967. The acts have been amended many times.

During the 1980s, as increasing evidence of the strong association between diet and health emerged, larger numbers of people began asking for changes in the nutrition-labeling law. Finally, the Nutrition Labeling and Education Act of 1990 (NLEA) was passed. This law required the federal government to participate in activities to educate consumers about use of the improved label information in making dietary choices. The NLEA has done much more. All products regulated by the FDA are required to have food labels. Since May 8, 1994, all packaged food must have labeling, and fresh fruits, vegetables, and seafood must have point-of-purchase information (information available about where the foods were purchased). Since July 6, 1994, the USDA requires nutrition labeling on packaged meat and poultry.

USE OF FOOD LABELS

While food labeling is useful for just about anyone, it may be of particular value to certain people, such as those who are trying to lose weight. The United States leads the world in obesity. In fact, about two-thirds of the U.S. population is now either overweight or obese. That is significantly higher than the 47 percent figure in the late 1970s.[11] A 2006 article in *Global Agenda* notes that in 1970 Americans spent about $6 billion at fast food chains; by 2005 that number had grown to $134 billion—much more than would be expected from inflation alone.[12] Still, it should be mentioned that many fast food chains, such as McDonald's, offer lower fat options, such as salads. But even when lower fat options are available, consumers may not purchase or eat them.

Food labels also are valuable for people trying to prevent cardiovascular problems. It is well known that higher intakes of saturated fat and cholesterol are correlated with elevated amounts of cholesterol in the blood. High blood cholesterol levels are, in turn, associated with a greater risk for coronary heart disease (CHD). The most common form of heart disease, CHD is a direct result of the narrowing of the arteries to the heart. The *Dietary Guidelines for Americans 2005*, which is updated every five years by the federally appointed Dietary Guidelines Advisory Committee, notes that daily fat intake should be between 20 and 35 percent of total calories. Most of these fat calories should come from polyunsaturated and monounsaturated sources, such as fish, nuts, and vegetable oils. (See chapter 4.) Intake of saturated fats should be restricted to less than 10 percent of calories and less than 300 milligrams per day of cholesterol. Trans fat consumption should be as low as possible.[13] If a product label states that it contains "partially hydrogenated" oils, it has trans fat.

A 2006 article in *Heart Advisor* stresses that consumers should make a point of checking the serving size. This is to "avoid a false sense of security."[14]

An interesting food labeling-related study was published in 2004 in *Social Science & Medicine*. Researchers examined the association between dietary intake of total fat, saturated fat, and cholesterol and the "search for total fat, saturated fat, and cholesterol information on food labels." As some might have predicted, people who consume higher amounts of total fat, saturated fat, and cholesterol are less likely to look for those fats on food labels. "These findings suggest encouraging search of food label information among consumers with unhealthy dietary habits would need innovative approaches."[15]

Similarly, people may wish to check labels to determine the amount of sodium. In some people, sodium has been found to raise blood pressure. High blood pressure is another risk factor for heart disease. The *Dietary Guidelines for Americans 2005* advises people to consume no more than 2,300 milligrams of sodium per day (approximately 1 teaspoon of salt). People who are already dealing with high blood pressure, as well as African American and middle-aged and older adults, should try to keep this number to 1,500 milligrams or lower.[16] Yet, according to a September 13, 2006 article in *The New York Times,* the average American now consumes more than 3,300 milligrams of sodium a day; that stands in contrast to the 3,100 milligrams that he or she consumed in 1994.[17] About three-quarters of this salt comes from processed foods. "No more than 10 percent comes out of the salt shaker, and another 10 percent is contained naturally in foods."[18]

Detecting sodium is not always easy. It is unseen in a number of foods, such as preservatives, flavorings, and stabilizers, and in kosher meats such as beef, lamb, and chicken. Sodium also is naturally present in foods like milk, cheese, meat, fish, and some vegetables.

A 2006 *Saturday Evening Post* article notes that one cup of canned soup may contain more than 50 percent of the recommended amount of daily salt, and a restaurant serving of lasagna may have more salt than one should be consuming in an entire day.[19]

CONTROVERSIES SURROUNDING FOOD LABELING

Although food labeling has many supporters, it has generated some controversy. Today, much of this revolves around the federal government's unwillingness to require labeling of genetically modified foods. (See chapter 8.) But there are also a few additional issues. One of the most common problems occurs when consumers misunderstand or misinterpret food labels. For example, if the label on a bottle of corn oil indicates that the product is free of cholesterol, consumers may conclude, incorrectly, that other brands of corn oil contain cholesterol. Corn oil is a plant-based food, and cholesterol is only found in animal-based foods. More accurate labeling would indicate that all corn oil is free of cholesterol, but advertisers always want their products to stand apart from the crowd. So a little fudging of the truth is not uncommon.

Food labels also tend to make the food appear more visually appealing than it actually is. Moreover, according to a 2007 article in *The Nation's Health*, a study released by the California-based Strategic Alliance for Healthy Food and Activity found that "more than half of all food products marketed to children that prominently feature fruit on their packaging contain no fruit at all." The study included a total of 37 products.[20]

On occasion, a food label may be incorrect. A 1999 story in *Family Practice News* reported that there have been at least three children who had life-threatening anaphylactic reactions to dark chocolate with "pareve" labeling, a kosher designation that means, in part, the absence of milk. The children experienced a number of serious reactions, such as coughing, congestion, asthma, hives, itching, angioedema, bronchospasm, diarrhea, vomiting, wheezing, and nonresponsiveness. All were transported to medical facilities to receive emergency treatment with epinephrine. The child who was nonresponsive required intubation. "The reason milk can be present in dark chocolate certified to be made without milk is that it is made on the same processing equipment as milk chocolate."[21] Cross-contamination obviously occurred.

Cross-contamination is a worry for people with celiac disease, an autoimmune disorder. Celiacs are unable to eat wheat, oats, barley, and rye. Although the ingredients in a corn cereal, as noted on the label, may be perfectly safe, if the cereal is processed on the same machinery as the gluten-containing cereals, there may well be cross-contamination. Celiacs often check directly with manufacturers to determine if the food is safe for them to eat. In *Kids with Celiac Disease*, which was published on 2001, Danna Korn writes that celiacs need to become good food label readers. If any of the following foods appear on an ingredient, the food may contain gluten:

- Brown rice syrup (frequently made from barley)
- Caramel color
- Dextrin (usually corn, but sometimes derived from wheat)
- Flour or cereal products

- Hydrolyzed vegetable protein (HVP), vegetable protein hydrolyzed plant protein (HPP), or textured vegetable protein (TVP)
- Malt or malt flavoring (usually made from barley; okay if made from corn)
- Malt vinegar
- Modified food starch or modified starch from an unspecified or forbidden source
- Mono- and diglycerides (in dry products)
- Flavorings in meat products
- Soy sauce or soy sauce solids (many soy sauces contain wheat)
- Vegetable gum[22]

In the book *Celiac Disease*, which was published in 2007, Sylvia Llewelyn Bower, Mary Kay Sharrett, and Steve Plogsted write that the following foods are safe for celiacs: amaranth, arrowroot, bean, bean flour, buckwheat, corn, flax, Indian rice grass, legumes, lentils, mesquite, millet, montina, nuts, potato, quinoa, rice, sorghum, soy, tapioca, teff, and wild rice. "However, all these grains and starches may become contaminated during the milling and manufacturing process, so it is important to purchase them from manufacturers who take precautions to eliminate cross-contamination."[23]

Furthermore, there is the issue of food labels that fail to tell the whole story. For example, if they fulfill the requirements and pay the fees, foods that are low in fat and saturated fat may include the "heart-check mark" on their labels. But, foods that are low in fat and saturated fat are not, necessarily, healthy. In fact, one of the approved foods, Chocolate Lucky Charms, contains a huge amount of sugar. No one needs to consume such high amounts of sugar, especially in a food that may be consumed on a daily basis.

Food labels have the potential to be confusing. The FDA requires that all labeling be "truthful and not misleading," but the FDA cannot monitor all products and cannot stop marketers from slightly bending the rules. In a 2001 article in *The New York Times*, Marian Burros wrote that she enjoys reading egg cartons. The label of one carton noted that the hens are "cage-free." Burros wondered what that really meant. Are the chickens free-range? Or are they not in cages, "but in large enclosed areas where they stand beak to beak"? One of Burros' favorite labels is used by a chicken producer who indicates that his birds have "no artificial hormones." Commenting on the label, Burros wrote, "A double asterisk beside the statement leads to this notice: 'USDA regulations prohibit the use of artificial growth stimulates and hormones in this product.' The company is making a virtue out of not doing what it is not permitted to do."[24]

In *Eating Between the Lines*, which was published in 2007, Kimberly Lord Stewart writes, "We'd all like to believe that 'free-range' means that hens spend the day basking in the sun, roaming in the grass, and clustering around Grandma's feet as she throws handfuls of Nebraska-grown corn from her apron pockets, but no such luck. The hens may have access to the outdoors, but they may actually never venture out the barn door. Most hens like to stay close to their nests, food, and water."[25]

A 2007 article in *Newsweek* explained that some of the terms used on labels may not be as clear as they should be. For example, a label may read "antibiotic free." That may not mean that the animal was never given any antibiotics. Rather, it may indicate that there were no antibiotics in the animal's system before slaughter. So consumers looking for antibiotic-free products should look for labels that say "raised without antibiotics." Another confusing term is "grass fed." Cows are often fed grass before being switched to grain, even on conventional farms. Animals fed grain are more prone to health problems that require antibiotics. Whenever possible, consumers should search for cows fed 99 percent grain.[26]

A study published in 2007 in *The Journal of Allergy and Clinical Immunology* noted that some consumers who should be reading labels very closely are not. Researchers studied whether consumers with peanut allergies were heeding the advice of advisory labeling. Such labeling indicates that the product may contain peanut allergen. Yet, although exposure to such an allergen may be deadly, consumers "are increasingly ignoring advisory labeling."[27] Ignoring the label does not remove the risk. "Because food products with advisory labeling do contain detectable levels of peanuts, a risk exists to consumers choosing to eat such foods."[28]

An interesting 2007 article in *Environmental Nutrition* discusses what all consumers should look for on food labels. First, look at serving sizes. They may vary widely from product to product. "Don't assume a small package equals one serving." Check for saturated and trans fat. It is better to consume foods with fewer than two grams of saturated fat and no trans fat. Though fiber is a very important part of the diet, many people eat far too little. A daily intake of around 25 grams is best. Watch the sodium—as previously noted, no more than 2,300 milligrams. Less is better. Because sugar has only empty calories, a reduced consumption is preferred.[29]

The article also advised consumers to look for three "red flags" on food labels. The first is "trans-fat-free." Just because a product is free of trans fats, it is not, necessarily healthful. The trans fats may be replaced with other fats that are high in saturated fat. The second term includes words like "wholesome, pure, and natural." The article maintains that these words mean "nothing." The federal government defines wholesome as "fit for human consumption," and pure and natural have no official definitions. The third red flag is "less or reduced sugar." That probably indicates that the product contains artificial sweetener. Just because a product has reduced amounts of sugar, it is not, necessarily, lower in calories. "Often, sugar-free or reduced-sugar foods have as many or even more calories than the originals."[30]

The author of the article concludes that, "Reading food labels may prolong grocery shopping trips, but if you're concerned about your health, it's well worth the time. Practice makes perfect; the more you work at it, the better—and faster—you'll get."[31]

CONCLUSION

It is becoming increasingly evident that many people are concerned about what is in the food that they eat. How much fat does it contain? Cholesterol? Sodium? This is important information, especially if someone has medical problems. One of the most obvious ways to learn what is in the food is to read food labels. Still, large numbers of people rarely do or never bother. Furthermore, not everyone supports the current labeling requirements. Some believe they are often confusing, misleading, or inaccurate.

TOPICS FOR DISCUSSION

1. Do you read food labels? Why or why not?
2. If you do read labels, what are you looking for? Why?
3. If you were developing food and nutrition labels for a box of cereal, what would you include? What would you delete? Why?
4. Has a food label ever caused you to purchase a product? Describe the experience. What triggered the sale?
5. Do you think that food labels are overcrowded with information? Why or why not?

NOTES

1. Thomas Philipson, "Government Perspective: Food Labeling," *American Journal of Clinical Nutrition* (July 2005) 82: 262S–4S.

2. Susan Borra, "Consumer Perspectives on Food Labels," *American Journal of Clinical Nutrition* (May 2006) 83: 1235S.

3. International Food Information Council website, http://www.ific.org.

4. Jonathan L. Blitstein and W. Douglas Evans, "Use of Nutrition Facts Among Adults Who Make Household Food Purchasing Decisions," *Journal of Nutrition Education and Behavior* (November—December 2006) 38: 360–364.

5. International Food Information Council website.

6. International Food Information Council website.

7. Richard Dahl, "Allergen Labeling Takes Effect," *Environmental Health Perspectives* (January 2006) 114: A24.

8. Linda Bren, "Food Labels Identify Allergens More Clearly," *FDA Consumer* (March-April 2006) 40: NA.

9. Center for Food Safety and Applied Nutrition, Food and Drug Administration website, http://www.cfsan.fda.gov.

10. Becky Gillette, "New Labeling Helps People Choose Foods Healthier for Heart," *Mississippi Business Journal* (January 30, 2006) 28: B4.

11. "Food Firms and Fat-Fighting; Food Companies and Obesity; It's All on the Label, So Don't Blame Us if It Makes You Fat," *Global Agenda* (February 9, 2006) NA.

12. "Food Firms and Fat-Fighting; Food Companies and Obesity; It's All on the Label, So Don't Blame Us if It Makes You Fat," NA.

13. http://www.health.gov/dietaryguidelines/dga2005/report.

14. "Cracking the Food Label Codes: For the Sake of Your Heart, Develop the Fine Art of Reading the Fine Print," *Heart Advisor* (October 2006) 9: 10.

15. Chung-Tung Jordan Lin, Jonq-Ying Lee, and Steven T. Yen, "Do Dietary Intakes Affect Search for Nutrient Information on Food Labels?" *Social Science & Medicine* (November 2004) 59: 1955–1967.

16. http://www.health.gov/dietaryguidelines/dga2005/report.

17. Melanie Warner, "The War Over Salt," *InsideNYTimes.com* (September 13, 2006).

18. Melanie Warner, "The War Over Salt."

19. "Warning: High-Salt Food," *Saturday Evening Post* (November—December 2006) 278: 20.

20. Donya C. Arias, "Many Kid Food Products with Fruit on the Label Contain No Real Fruit," *The Nation's Health* (April 2007) 37: 16.

21. Sharon Worcester, "Pareve Labeling Doesn't Always Mean Milk Free," *Family Practice News* (May 1, 1999) 29: 54.

22. Danna Korn, *Kids with Celiac Disease* (Bethesda, Maryland: Woodbine House, 2001).

23. Sylvia Llewelyn Bower, *Celiac Disease* (New York: Demos Medical Publishing, 2007) 28.

24. Marian Burros, "Eating Well: The Truth Behind the Feel-Good Labels," *The New York Times* (March 14, 2001) Section F, Page 2, Column 1.

25. Kimberly Lord Stewart, *Eating Between the Lines* (New York: St. Martin's Griffin, 2007) 88.

26. Anna Kuchment, "What's On Your Label?" *Newsweek* (March 12. 2007) 63.

27. Susan L. Hefle, Terence J. Furlong, Lynn Niemann, et al., "Consumer Attitudes and Risks Associated with Packaged Foods Having Advisory Labeling Regarding the Presence of Peanuts," *The Journal of Allergy and Clinical Immunology* (July 2007) 120: 171–6.

28. Susan L. Hefle, Terence J. Furlong, Lynn Niemann, et al. "Consumer Attitudes and Risks Associated with Packaged Foods Having Advisory Labeling Regarding the Presence of Peanuts," 171–6.

29. Diane Welland, "Red-Flagging Food Labels: 8 Tips to Sift Fact from Fiction," *Environmental Nutrition* (March 2007) 30: 2.

30. Diane Wellard, "Red-Flagging Food Labels: 8 Tips to Sift Fact from Fiction," 2.

31. Diane Wellard, "Red-Flagging Food Labels: 8 Tips to Sift Fact from Fiction," 2.

REFERENCES AND RESOURCES

Books

Korn, Danna. *Kids with Celiac Disease.* Bethesda, Maryland: Woodbine House, 2001.
Llewelyn Bower, Sylvia with Mary Kay Sharrett and Steve Plogsted. *Celiac Disease.* New York: Demos Medical Publishing, 2007.
Lord Stewart, Kimberley. *Eating Between the Lines.* New York: St. Martin's Griffin, 2007.

Magazines, Journals, and Newspapers

Arias, Donya C. "Many Kid Food Products with Fruit on the Label Contain No Real Fruit." *The Nation's Health* (April 2007) 37: 16.
Blitstein, Jonathan and W. Douglas Evans. "Use of Nutrition Facts Panels Among Adults Who Make Household Food Purchasing Decisions." *Journal of Nutrition Education and Behavior* (November—December 2006) 38: 360–4.
Borra, Susan. "Consumers Perspectives on Food Labels." *American Journal of Clinical Nutrition* (May 2006) 83: 1235S.
Bren, Linda. "Food Labels Identify Allergens More Clearly." *FDA Consumer* (March—April 2006) 40: NA.
Burros, Marian. "Eating Well: The Truth Behind the Feel-Good-Labels." *The New York Times* (March 14, 2001) Section F, Page 2, Column 1.
"Cracking the Food Label Codes: For the Sake of Your Heart, Develop the Fine Art of Reading the Fine Print." *Heart Advisor* (October 2006) 9: 10.
Dahl, Richard. "Allergen Labeling Takes Effects." *Environmental Health Perspectives* (January 2006) 114: A24.
"Food Firms and Fat-Fighters; Food Companies and Obesity; It's All on the Label, So Don't Blame Us If It Makes You Fat." *Global Agenda* (February 9, 2006) NA.
Gillette, Becky. "New Labeling Helps People Choose Foods Healthier for Heart." *Mississippi Business Journal* (January 30, 2006) 28: B4.
Hefle, Susan L., Terence J. Furlong, Lynn Niemann, et al. "Consumer Attitudes and Risks Associated with Package Foods Having Advisory Labeling Regarding the Presence of Peanuts." *The Journal of Allergy and Clinical Immunology* (July 2007) 120: 171–6.
Kuchment, Anna. "What's On Your Label?" *Newsweek* (March 12, 2007) 63.
Lin, Chung-Tung Jordan, Jonq-Ying Lee, and Steven T. Yen. "Do Dietary Intakes Affect Search for Nutrient Information on Food Labels?" *Social Science & Medicine* (November 2004) 59: 1955–67.
Philipson, Tomas. "Government Perspective: Food Labeling." *American Journal of Clinical Nutrition* (July 2005) 82: 262S–4S.
Warner, Melanie. "The War Over Salt." *InsideNYTimes.com* (September 13, 2006).

"Warning: High-Salt Food." *Saturday Evening Post* (November—December 2006) 278: 20.

Welland, Diane. "Red-Flagging Food Labels: 8 Tips to Sift Fact from Fiction." *Environmental Nutrition* (March 2007) 30: 2.

Worcester, Sharon. "Pareve Labeling Doesn't Always Mean Milk Free." *Family Practice News* (May 1, 1999) 29: 54.

Websites

American Heart Association
http://www.americanheart.org

Center for Food Safety and Applied Nutrition, Food and Drug Administration
http://www.cfsan.fda.gov

International Food Information Council
http://www.ific.org

U.S. Department of Agriculture
http://www.usda.gov

Chapter 7

Genetically Engineered Dairy Products

Who can resist? A tall glass of milk goes so well with a chocolate chip cookie.

A big bowl of ice cream is a perfect ending to that celebratory dinner. And smooth cream cheese glides so effortlessly over that toasted bagel. Just talking about these foods makes the mouth water. But they might also be reason for concern.

Some of the dairy products sold in the United States are produced with the assistance of the genetically engineered synthetic animal growth hormone known as recombinant bovine somatotropin (rBST) or recombinant bovine growth hormone (rBGH). The product, which was developed by the St. Louis-based giant corporation Monsanto and sold with the brand name Posilac, was approved by the U.S. Food and Drug Administration in November 1993. Commercially available since 1994, Posilac, which is injected into cows, boosts the production of milk. However, for years there has been ongoing controversy about whether this hormone is safe or if it is putting the welfare and well-being of both consumers and cows at risk.

Avoiding the use of the word hormone, supporters of this product often refer to it as recombinant bovine somatotropin or bovine somatotropin (rBST or bST); those who are opposed to this product tend to include hormone in the name and to refer to it as recombinant bovine growth hormone. (But these terms may also be used interchangeably.) In this chapter, when not part of a quote, it will be called Posilac or rBST/rBGH, a combination of both names.

ARGUMENTS FOR THE SAFETY OF POSILAC

No one should be surprised that Monsanto insists that rBST/rBGH, or as Monsanto notes bST or Posilac, is safe. In fact, Monsanto says

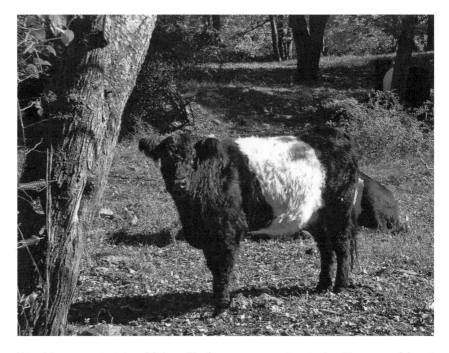

Would you want to drink milk from a cow treated with recombinant bovine growth hormone? (Courtesy of Mark A. Goldstein)

that, "Milk from cows receiving supplemental bST is unchanged and just as wholesome and nutritious as always—full of calcium, protein, phosphorous and vitamins.... Research has shown that cows given supplemental bST in the form of Posilac become more efficient milk producers, without jeopardizing milk quality, animal health, or wholesomeness in the process."[1]

Because Posilac enables farmers to produce more milk with fewer cows, Mosanto adds that Posilac has some additional benefits. For every 1 million dairy cows that receive Posilac supplementation, there is an annual saving of 6.6 billion gallons of water, a 3 billion reduction in the amount of animal feed needed, a decrease in the need for over 417 square miles of land, a savings of 5.5 million gallons of gasoline, a lowering of greenhouse gases by 30,000 metric tons, and manure reduction of about 3.6 million tons.[2]

While denying that Posilac causes any problems in humans, Monsanto does admit that it has the potential to compromise the health of cows. The label warns of mastitis (requiring antibiotic treatment), digestive disorders, lameness, hoof problems, increased physical stress and resulting shortening of life, problems with metabolism, and greater chance of multiple births.[3]

Since approving rBST/rBGH, the U.S. Food and Drug Administration has consistently and repeatedly stated that it is safe. Over and over again, in different reports and in responses to many challenges, the FDA has said essentially the same thing. "The FDA believes that the available data confirm that biologically significant amounts of rBGH are not absorbed in humans following the consumption of milk from cows treated with rBGH."[4] Even when it is not digested, according to Monsanto, rBST/rBGH is too large to pass through the wall of the gut. And what happens when it is administered intravenously? Nothing. There "was no activity in humans."[5]

The American Council on Science and Health (ACSH) notes that several well-respected organizations support the use of rBST/rBGH. For example, ACSH indicates that the American Medical Association says that bovine somatotropin is "a hormone that is produced naturally by cows to help them make milk." Supplementing cows with rBST/rBGH allows them to produce between 10 and 40 percent more milk. This is accomplished without "harming the animal or altering the nutritional value of the milk."[6]

Similarly, ACSH observes that the American Cancer Society says that "there are no valid findings to indicate a risk of human carcinogenesis." The Children's Nutrition Research Center at Baylor College of Medicine says that if these claims against rBST/rBGH were valid, "then human colostrum, human breast milk, and indeed, all milk would be incriminated as a cause of cancer—women and their children have nothing to fear regarding the nation's milk supply."[7]

Some of the sharpest criticism comes from former U. S. Surgeon General C. Everett Koop. He contends that a "few fringe groups are using misleading statements and blatant falsehoods" to scare consumers, thereby preventing them from benefiting from biotechnological advances. "Because diary foods are an important, widely consumed source of nutrition, it is necessary to condemn these attacks on the safety of milk for what they are: baseless, manipulative and completely irresponsible."[8]

To ACSH, spending extra for organic milk or ice cream, which do not contain rBST/rBGH, is simply a waste of money. Because dairy cows produce bovine growth hormones, all types of milk contain them. Supplementation with rBST/rBGH "does not change the milk in any way."[9] Thomas G. Baumgartner, a University of Florida clinical professor in the colleges of medicine, pharmacy, and dentistry who also serves on the American Council on Science and Health, acknowledges that "synthetic hormones from milk could spawn serious problems—including cancer—if introduced to the bloodstream," but stomach acids "break down the potentially harmful elements before they can be absorbed." According to Baumgartner, "there is not a spattering of evidence that there's any harm in drinking regular milk."[10]

The ACSH admits that rBST/rBGH does increase the hormone known as insulin growth factor (IGF-1) in milk. When IGF-1 is produced by the body, it may lead to hypertension, cancers, and other medical problems. But the ACSH says that increasing amounts of IGF-1 in milk is not a concern. "Any hormonal activity is destroyed as the IGF-1 is digested."[11]

ARGUMENTS AGAINST THE USE OF POSILAC

Not everyone is supportive of Posilac. In fact, growing numbers of people are demanding that farmers stop using it. Much of the soaring sales of organic milk is directly attributable to fears associated with milk from cows treated with rBST/rBGH.

It is important to go back to the beginning. Before approval by the FDA, from 1986 until 1990, Posilac underwent trials at the University of Vermont. During that time Andrew Christiansen, a state representative and dairy farmer from East Montpelier, spread the word about the treated cows experiencing health problems and giving birth to deformed calves. Bernard Sanders, Vermont's U.S. representative, asked the General Accounting Office to investigate. "In its report, the GAO faulted the FDA—with many former Monsanto employees in key positions—for using guidelines that did not fully address food-safety risks."[12] Yet Congress took no action to delay approval.

An article on the website of the Council for Responsible Genetics outlines aspects of the less than pristine method in which Posilac was approved. The article, entitled "Whistleblowers, Threats, and Bribes," explains that an FDA veterinarian named Richard Burroughs, one of the supervisors of the Posilac review process, expressed concern that the agency was ordering an inadequate number of tests. When Burroughs ordered more tests, he was told he was slowing the approval process and was fired. Alexander Apostolou, the director of the FDA's Division of Toxicology, also voiced his concern, and he was asked to leave. Then, after testifying that there was "a systematic human food safety breakdown at the Center for Veterinary Medicine [at the FDA]," Joseph Settepani, a supervising chemist, was demoted.[13]

A 2006 article in *Townsend Letter: The Examiner of Alternative Medicine* notes a few additional reasons for concern. Margaret Miller, the researcher at Monsanto who developed rBST/rBGH, was hired by the FDA "to oversee the review process of the genetically engineered drug." When she completed the job, she returned to Monsanto.[14]

A 1999 article in *The Nation* explains that Michael Taylor, a former Monsanto attorney who became FDA deputy commissioner for policy, decided that since "rBGH is not an additive," it need not be listed on product labels.[15] A few years after completing his work at the FDA, Taylor returned to Monsanto, as a vice-president. The organization

Sustainable Table, a group that educates consumers about food-related issues, refers to a "revolving door" between the FDA and Monsanto.[16]

Whatever happened or didn't happen at the FDA and Monsanto, people who are worried about rBST/rBGH tend to focus less on the "revolving door" and the ethical questions that it raises and more on safety issues. Specifically, is it safe to consume dairy products obtained from cows who have been treated with rBST/rBGH?

As has previously been noted, supporters of the use of rBST/rBGH agree that it contributes to the body's production of higher amounts of insulin growth factor (IGF-1), which may compromise health. But they stress that hormonal activity is killed during digestion. People who oppose the use of rBST/rBGH are not so sure that is true. They also note that "both the European Union and Canada have banned rBGH due to safety concerns."[17] In addition, rBST/rBGH is banned in Australia, New Zealand, and Japan. Furthermore, they frequently cite the belief that rBST/rBGH was never properly tested before it was approved. According to Sustainable Table, "the FDA relied solely on a study done by Monsanto in which rBGH was tested for 90 days on 30 rats. The study was never published, and the FDA stated the result showed no significant problems. But a review by the Canadian health agency [Health Canada—equivalent to the FDA] on rBGH found the 90 day study showed a significant number of issues which should have triggered a full review by the FDA."[18]

Michael Hansen, a researcher with Consumer Policy Institute, Consumer Union, commented on these "issues." He said that when Health Canada reviewed the entire study, it learned that "20 to 30 percent of the rats in the high dose group developed primary antibody responses to rBGH, suggesting it was being absorbed into the bloodstream." Some of the male rats also had cysts on their thyroid glands.[19]

One of the most longstanding and vocal opponents of rBST/rBGH is Samuel S. Epstein, a professor emeritus of environmental medicine at the University of Illinois at Chicago School of Public Health. His organization, Cancer Prevention Coalition, lists the following reasons to avoid dairy products with rBST/rBGH:

- rBGH makes cows sick. Monsanto has been forced to admit to 20 basic toxic effects, including mastitis, on its Posilac label.
- rBGH milk is contaminated by pus, due to the mastitis commonly induced by rBGH, and antibiotics to treat mastitis.
- rBGH milk is chemically and nutritionally different than natural milk.
- rBGH milk is contaminated with rBGH, traces of which are absorbed through the gut.
- rBGH milk is supercharged with high levels of a natural growth factor (IGF-1), which is readily absorbed through the gut.

- Excess levels of IGF-1 have been incriminated as a cause of breast, colon, and prostate cancer.
- IGF-1 blocks natural defense mechanisms against early submicroscopic cancers.
- rBGH factory farms pose a major threat to the viability of small dairy farms.
- rBGH enriches Monsanto, while posing dangers, without any benefits, to consumers, especially in view of the current national surplus of milk.[20]

When a May 2006 article in *The Journal of Reproductive Medicine* noted that vegetarian and omnivore women have a twinning rate five times higher than vegan women, Epstein commented in "Hormonal Milk Poses Greater Risks Than Just Twinning," which was published in June 2006 in Ascribe: The Public Interest Newswire, that these results were not surprising. "Hormonal milk contains up to ten-fold increased levels of the natural insulin-like growth factor, known as IGF, long known to increase ovulation and twinning rates in cows."[21]

But instead of worry about twinning, Epstein is far more concerned about the association between rBST/rBGH and cancer, especially in children, "in view of their high susceptibility to cancer-causing products and chemicals." He also expresses regrets that all too few schools make organic milk available to their students.[22]

An article published in 2003 in the *Townsend Letter for Doctors and Patients* noted that every year, Americans consume almost 180 billion pounds of milk products. That means, on average, each year a typical American eats about 666 pounds of milk products. For most Americans at least some of these milk products come from cows treated with rBST/rBGH. So they contain higher levels of IGF-1. According to the author, the casein in the milk as well as the homogenization process facilitates the passage of the hormone into the bloodstream. Because IGF-1 is known to accelerate cancer growth, researchers have found a direct association between high levels of IGF-1 and pancreatic cancer cells, endometrial tumor cells, central nervous system tumor, primary colorectal tumors, thyroid papillary cancer cells, and bone tumors, specifically osteogenic sarcoma. Moreover, researchers have found a four-fold increased risk of prostate cancer in men with the highest levels of IGF-1.[23] In a study on the relationship between IGF-1 and breast cancer, "after adjusting for known breast cancer factors (including age at onset of menarche, number of children, age at birth of first child and family history), the study did find a seven fold increased risk of breast cancer among pre-menopausal women less than 51 years of age with the highest relative levels of IGF-1 identified in their blood."[24]

Over the years researchers continued to study the potential problems associated with the use of rBST/rBGH, periodically waving red flags. In a 2000 editorial in the *British Medical Journal*, three researchers noted that it has been proven that people with elevated rates of IGF-1 have higher rates of cancer. Thus, in animals, it has been found that calorie restriction lowers the rates of cancer because it reduces the amount of circulating IGF-1. As a result, the researchers stress that, "given the increasing evidence of the risk of cancer, caution should be exercised in the exogenous use of either insulin-like growth factor-1 or substances that increase concentrations of it."[25]

That same year an article published in the *Journal of the National Cancer Institute* said that in laboratory studies it was determined that IGF-1 transforms cells and prevents cell death. The authors conclude that "the role of IGF-1 in cancer is supported by epidemiologic studies which have found high levels of circulating IGF-1 ... are associated with increased risk of several common cancers ..."[26]

Similar opinions were expressed in a 2002 article published in *Oncology*. Two researchers noted, "a growing number of epidemiologic studies suggest that increased serum levels of IGFs and/or altered levels of their binding proteins are associated with increased risk for developing several malignancies."[27]

Another study from 2002, which was published in the *International Journal of Cancer,* examined the relationship between high circulation IGF-1 concentrations and increased risk of ovarian cancer. Included in the study were 132 women with primary invasive epithelial ovarian cancer. For each of these women, there were two control subjects. Again, the researchers found "a strong direct relationship between circulating IGF-1 levels and risk of developing ovarian cancer before age 55."[28]

A 2004 study published in the *Journal of Clinical Oncology* evaluated the relationship between circulating IGF-1 levels in 281 men who were diagnosed with prostate cancer after recruitment and 560 matched controls. Researchers concluded that their "data add further support for IGF-1 as an etiologic factor in prostate cancer and indicate that circulating IGF-1 levels ... may be most strongly associated with prostate cancer risk."[29]

As the years have passed, a number of individuals and nonprofit groups have kept the anti-rBST/rBGH message alive. One of these is the Physicians for Social Responsibility, Oregon Chapter. As part of their Campaign for Safe Food, representatives of this group have given many presentations on the topic of rBST/rBGH. The group believes that if more consumers learned the truth about rBST/rBGH, they will stop purchasing dairy products from treated cows. If this were to occur, dairy farmers would have no incentive to use it. Their website (**http://oregonpsr.org**) contains a brochure, "Know Your Milk" as well as information on rBGH/rBST-free dairy products. A February 21, 2007, press release issued by the Organic Consumers Association notes that the "Oregon Physicians for Social Responsibility has made nearly

150 presentations giving both sides on rBGH to all kinds of audiences—mothers' clubs, school boards, businesses, Rotary clubs, church groups, college, neighborhoods etc. If there is one constant we've found, it's this: The more people know about rBGH, the more they avoid it."[30]

So it should not be surprising that sales of organic milk have risen by about 25 percent a year; more recently, sales of milk from untreated cows has also been rising, "even as overall milk sales remain flat."[31] (Organic milk costs about twice the price of regular milk. Milk that is free of rBST/rBGH costs about 10–15 percent more than regular milk.) Consumers are increasingly gravitating to milk that is labeled "rBST-free" or "rBGH-free." (Because all milk contains hormones, companies are unable to label or advertise their milk as "hormone free.") A 2006 article in *Feedstuffs* describes a newspaper story in which a mother who is shopping for her family selects string cheese because the label notes that it does not contain bST. The mother is then quoted as follows: "I'm not sure what it is, but I think it is something bad. I'm pretty certain it's a hormone, and I try to buy milk that also doesn't have hormones in it. I'm not one of those people where everything has to be organic, but with my child, I feel like I should get her off on the right food—you know, without pesticides and hormones."[32]

In a September 2006 article printed in *St. Paul Pioneer Press*, Ann Mayer, a mother of two-year-old Luke, says, though she isn't very "choosy" about what she eats, she is careful what Luke eats, even if she needs to pay more. "Mayer chooses organic foods for her toddler, and buys both organic milk and conventional Land O'Lakes milk from cows not treated with rBST. 'I just won't buy the other stuff,' she said. 'Luckily, these days, you don't have to go too far out of the way to do it.'"[33]

In fact, in recent years r-BST-free or rBGH-free labels have become a marketing tool. For example, in April 2007, Publix Super Markets Inc., which is based in Lakeland, Florida, announced that its private label milk would no longer contain rBST/rBGH. Shannon Patten, a Publix spokeswoman, said that, "When it comes to our decision to carry rBST-free milk, we are simply listening and responding to what our customers have asked for.[34] Publix has about 900 stores in the South."[35] Following that action, Southeast Milk Inc., Florida's largest dairy cooperative, decided to cease using rBST/rBGH on its farms by September 1, 2007.

But this trend is not only confined to the southern portion of the country. In 2007 "The Organic & Non-GMO Report" noted that "Dean Foods, the nation's largest dairy processor, has converted to rBGH-free production in several of its New England facilities, and grocery giant Safeway has done the same in Washington and Oregon."[36]

By the end of 2007 Starbucks stores throughout the country used only rBST/rBGH-free dairy products. That represents about 32 million gallons of milk per year.[37] And, with over 530 restaurants, the Denver-based Chipotle Mexican Grill serves only rBST/rBGH-free sour cream and cheese. Some locations offer only rBST/rBGH-free organic milk. Steve Ells, the founder, chairman, and CEO of Chipotle Mexican Grill, said, "We want to change the way the world thinks about and eats fast food. Serving our customers cheese and sour cream without rBGH is the responsible thing to do. It's better for our customers, better for the animals, and better for the food system."[38]

As of February 2008 food industry giant Kroger sold only rBST/rBGH-free milk. Food & Water Watch notes that increasing numbers of businesses, college campuses, and hospitals are purchasing rBST/rBGH-free milk. According to the ENN Environmental New Network, "the number of dairies using the hormone is falling like dominoes across the country."[39]

And, increasingly, consumers want labels to indicate if dairy products have been produced without the use of rBST/rBGH. From February 28, 2007, through March 5, 2007, Lake Research Partners conducted a survey of 1,000 adults living in private households in the continental United States. The following statement was read to survey participants: "Some milk comes from cows that have been treated with an artificial growth hormone called rBGH to increase their milk production. Other milk comes from cows that have not been treated with the hormones. Some people want to label dairy products according to whether or not they are from cows that have been treated with rBGH. What do you think? Should milk from cows that have not been treated with the hormone rBGH be allowed to be labeled as 'rBGH free,' or should that not be allowed?"[40] Eighty percent of the participants indicated that they preferred that the milk be labeled rBGH-free; fifteen percent preferred no labeling; five percent didn't know.[41]

Meanwhile, Monsanto continues to insist that there is no difference in milk obtained with or without the use of rBST/rBGH. (Technically, that is not true. Posilac adds one amino acid—methionine—to the cow's natural growth hormone.[42]) Monsanto claims that those who use rBST/rBGH-free labeling delude consumers into thinking milk produced without using hormones is healthier and safer.

Though the battle between Monsanto and those who wish to use the rBST/rBGH-free labels shows no sign of abating, it is significant to note that in the middle of 2007 the Federal Trade Commission refused to stop dairies and companies from advertising their milk as free from synthetic hormones. In 2007, Mosanto announced that its profits from Posilac were 16 percent less than the previous year.[43]

In August 2008, Monsanto announced plans to sell Posilac to Elanco, the animal health division of Eli Lily and Company. A press release issued by Monsanto stated that, "Lily will purchase assets and liabilities of Monsanto associated with the POSILAC brand and related business for an upfront payment of $300 million, plus additional contingent consideration." The press release also noted that, "Over the past 14 years, more than a half billion units of POSILAC have been successfully and safely used by tens of thousands of dairy producers on millions of cows to produce wholesome, nutritious, safe and affordable milk and dairy products."[44]

CONCLUSION

It is quite evident that the U.S. Food and Drug Administration, as well as many well respected organizations and individuals, insist that milk and milk products derived from cows treated with Posilac is safe. They maintain that the milk is the same as milk obtained from cows not treated with Posilac. So, according to them, there is absolutely no reason to pay the extra cost associated with milk from cows not treated with Posilac or organic milk.

Many consumers still are not convinced. They worry that consuming milk or milk products from Posilac-treated cows may have long-term negative consequences, especially to their children. To them, it is important to obtain milk and milk products from untreated cows. The numbers of people refusing to consume milk products from treated cows keeps rising. If the trend continues, and dairy farmers have trouble selling their milk from treated cows, then the controversy will be settled by the marketplace. Farmers will have little incentive to produce milk they cannot sell.

NOTES

1. Monsanto website, http://www.monsanto.com.
2. Monsanto website.
3. Rose Marie Williams, "Bovine Growth Hormone: Consumers Fight Back," *Townsend Letter: The Examiner of Alternative Medicine* (April 2007) 285: 60–62.
4. U.S. Food and Drug Administration website, http://www.fda.gov.
5. Monsanto website.
6. American Council on Science and Health website, http:///www.acsh.org.
7. American Council on Science and Health website.
8. American Council on Science and Health website.
9. American Council on Science and Health website.
10. American Council on Science and Health website.
11. American Council on Science and Health website.
12. Daniel Bellow, "Vermont, the Pure-Food State: Vermont and Monsanto Co. Locked in Battle Over Use of Genetically Engineered Animal Hormone," *The Nation* (March 8, 1999) 268: 18.

13. Jeffrey Smith, "Whistleblowers, Threats and Bribes," Council for Responsible Genetics website, http://www.gene-watch.org.

14. Rose Marie Williams, "Bovine Growth Hormone Cover-Up," *Townsend Letter: The Examiner of Alternative Medicine* (November 2006) 280: 38–40.

15. Daniel Bellow, "Vermont, the Pure-Food State: Vermont and Monsanto Co. Locked in Battle Over Use of Genetically Engineered Animal Hormone."

16. Sustainable Table website, http://www.sustainable.org.

17. Sustainable Table website.

18. Sustainable Table website.

19. Consumers Union website, http://www.consumersunion.org.

20. Cancer Prevention Coalition website, http://www.preventcancer.com.

21. Samuel Epstein, "Hormonal Milk Poses Greater Risks than Just Twinning," Ascribe: The Public Interest Newswire website, http://www.ascribe.org.

22. Samuel Epstein, "Hormonal Milk Poses Greater Risks than Just Twinning."

23. Gina L. Nick, "Assessing Individual Susceptibility to Endocrine Disruption Caused by the Ingestion of Genetically Modified Organisms (GMOs). Part 1," *Townsend Letter for Doctors and Patients* (December 2003) 245: 116–7.

24. Gina L. Nick, "Assessing Individual Susceptibility to Endocrine Disruption Caused by the Ingestion of Genetically Modified Organisms (GMO) Part 1."

25. George Davey Smith, David Gunnell, and Jeff Holly. "Cancer and Insulin-Like Growth Factor-1." *British Medical Journal* (October 7, 2000) 321: 847–8.

26. Herbert Yu and Thomas Rohan, "Role of the Insulin-Like Growth Factor Family in Cancer Development and Progression," *Journal of the National Cancer Institute* (September 20, 2000) 92: 1472–89.

27. Stergios J. Moschos and Christos S. Mantzoros, "The Role of the IGF System in Cancer: From Basic to Clinical Studies and Clinical Applications." *Oncology* (November 2002) 63: 317–32.

28. Annekatrin Lukanova, Eva Lundin, Paolo Toniolo et al., "Circulating Levels of Insulin-Like Growth Factor-1 and Risk of Ovarian Cancer," *International Journal of Cancer* (August 2002) 101: 549–54.

29. Pär Stattin, Sabina Rinaldi, Carine Biessy et al., "High Levels of Circulating Insulin-Like Growth Factor-1 Increase Prostate Cancer Risk: A Prospective Study in a Population-based Nonscreened Cohort," *Journal of Clinical Oncology* (August 1, 2004) 22: 3104.

30. Organic Consumers Association website, http://www.organicconsumers.org.

31. Tom Webb, "New Parents Reach for BST-Free Milk," *St. Paul Pioneer Press* (MN) (September 23, 2006) NA.

32. Terry D. Etherton, "RbST-Free Milk—A Story of Smoke and Mirrors," *Feedstuffs* (October 9, 2006) 78: 9.

33. Tom Webb, "New Parents Reach for BST-Free Milk."

34. Kyle Kennedy, "Producers Dropping Production-Increasing Hormone," *The Ledger* (Lakeland, FL) (June 10, 2007) NA.

35. The Organic & Non-GMO Report website, http://www.non-gmoreport.com (September 2007).

36. The Organic & Non-GMO Report website (September 2007).

37. Organic Consumers Association website.

38. Organic Consumers Association website.

39. ENN Environmental News Network, http://www.enn.com.

40. Food & Water Watch website, www.foodandwaterwatch.org.

41. Food & Water Watch website.
42. Organic Consumers Association website.
43. ENN Environmental News Network website.
44. Monsanto website, http://www.Monsanto.com.

REFERENCES AND RESOURCES

Books

Epstein, Samuel S. *Cancer-Gate: How to Win the Losing Cancer War.* Amityville, New York: Baywood Publishing Company, Inc., 2005.
Smith, Jeffrey M. *Seeds of Deception.* Fairfield, Iowa: Yes! Books, 2003.

Magazines, Journals, and Newspapers

Bellow, Daniel. "Vermont, the Pure-Food State: Vermont and Monsanto Co. Locked in Battle Over Use of Genetically Engineered Animal Hormone." *The Nation* (March 8, 1999) 268: 18.
Etherton, Terry D. "RbST-Free Milk—A Story of Smoke and Mirrors." *Feedstuffs* (October 9, 2006) 78: 9.
Kennedy, Kyle. "Producers Dropping Production-Increasing Hormone." *The Ledger* (Lakeland, FL) (June 10, 2007) NA.
Lukanova, Annekatrin, Eva Lundin, Paolo Toniolo et al. "Circulating Levels of Insulin-Like Growth Factor-1 and Risk of Ovarian Cancer." *International Journal of Cancer* (August 2002) 101: 549—54.
Mohl, Bruce. "Stores Hike Prices On Milk Free of Synthetic Hormones." *Knight Ridder/ Tribune Business News* (October 10, 2006) NA.
Moschos, Stergios J. and Christos S. Mantzoros. "The Role of IGF System in Cancer: From Basic to Clinical Studies and Clinical Application." *Oncology* (November 2002) 63: 317–32.
Nick, Gina L. "Assessing Individual Susceptibility to Endocrine Disruption Caused by the Ingestion of Genetically Modified Organisms (GMOs). Part 1." *Townsend Letter for Doctors and Patients* (December 2003) 245: 116–7.
Smith, George Davey, David Gunnell, and Jeff Holly. "Cancer and Insulin-Like Growth Factor-1." *British Medical Journal* (October 7, 2000) 321: 847–8.
Stattin, Pär, Sabina Rinaldi, Carine Biessy et al. "High Levels of Circulating Insulin-Like Growth Factor-1 Increase Prostate Cancer Risk: A Prospective Study in a Population-Based Nonscreened Cohort." *Journal of Clinical Oncology* (August 1, 2004) 22: 3104–12.
Steinman, Gary. "Mechanisms of Twinning: VII. Effect of Diet and Heredity on the Human Twinning Rate." *The Journal of Reproductive Medicine* (May 2006) 51: 405–10.
Webb, Tom. "New Parents Reach for BST-Free Milk." *St. Paul Pioneer Press* (MN) (December 23, 2006) NA.
Williams, Rose Marie. "Bovine Growth Hormone: Consumers Fight Back." *Townsend Letter: The Examiner of Alternative Medicine* (April 2007) 285: 60–62.
Williams, Rose Marie. "Bovine Growth Hormones Cover-Up." *Townsend Letter: The Examiner of Alternative Medicine* (November 2006) 280: 38–40.

Yu, Herbert and Thomas Rohan. "Role of Insulin-Like Growth Factor in Cancer Development and Progression." *Journal of the National Cancer Institute* (September 20, 2000) 92(18): 1472–89.

Websites

American Council on Science and Health
http://www.acsh.org

AScribe: The Public Interest Newswire
http://www.ascribe.org

Cancer Prevention Coalition
http://www.preventcancer.com

Consumers Union
http://www.consumersunion.org

Council for Responsible Genetics
http://www.gene-watch.org

ENN Environmental News Network
http://www.enn.com

Food & Water Watch
www.foodandwaterwatch.org

HealthNewsDigest.com
http://healthnewsdigest.com

Monsanto
http://www.monsanto.com

Organic Consumers Association
http://www.organicconsumers.org

Physicians for Social Responsibility, Oregon Chapter
http://www.oregonpsr.org

Sustainable Table
http://www.sustainabletable.org

The Organic & Non-GMO Report
http://www.non-gmoreport.com

The Center for Food Safety
http://www.centerforfoodsafety.org

U. S. Food and Drug Administration
http://www.fda.gov

Chapter 8

Genetically Modified Foods

Increasingly, genetically modified foods are making their way to the marketplace. Because they are not labeled, consumers generally do not know that they are eating such products. Many people are not comfortable with the present system.

Not that long ago, one rarely heard about genetically modified organisms (GMOs), also known as genetically engineered crops. In fact, few people knew exactly what they were. That is no longer the case. GMOs, or plants, animals, or microorganisms that have been genetically altered or engineered for a specific purpose, are everywhere. The GEO-PIE Cooperative Extension Program of Cornell University estimates "that more than 60% of food products on U.S. shelves may contain at least some small quantity of some crop that has been genetically engineered."[1] So, how does a consumer determine which foods have been genetically modified. The program notes that people who consume foods containing non-organic corn, soybeans, and canola and cottonseed oils are probably eating genetically modified foods. Potatoes, squash, zucchini, and papayas may be genetically engineered, but generally are not.[2]

The International Service for the Acquisition of Agri-Biotech Applications, an international nonprofit that advocates for biotechnology, notes that in 2007 the use of biotech crops continued to rise. "Remarkably, growth continued at a sustained double-digit growth rate of 12%, or 12.3 million hectares (30 million acres)—the second highest increase in global biotech crop area in the last five years—reaching 114.3 million hectares (282.4 million acres).... In 2007, the number of countries planting biotech crops increased to 23, and comprised 12 developing countries and 11 industrial countries." Of these, the first ten countries, in order of hectarage, are U.S. (with 57.7 million hectares), Argentina, Brazil, Canada, India, China, Paraguay, South Africa, Uruguay, and the Philippines.[3]

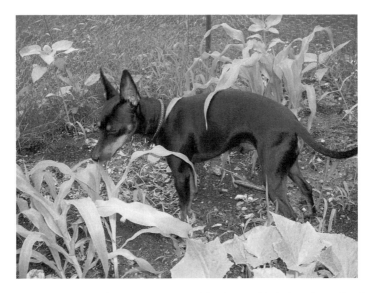

Even genetically modified corn should be knee high by the 4th of July. (Courtesy of Mark A. Goldstein)

In *Genetically Engineered Food: Changing the Nature of Nature*, which was published in 2001, Martin Teitel, president of the Council for Responsible Genetics, and Kimberly A. Wilson, former director of the Council's program on Commercial Biotechnology and the Environment, describe the sweeping changes brought about by GMOs. "The genetic engineering of our food is the most radical transformation in our diet since the invention of agriculture 10,000 years ago. . . . In the new kind of agriculture, a handful of giant corporations have placed patents on food plants, giving them exclusive control over that food. These transnational corporations have altered the ... life-processes of food plants by removing or adding genetic material in ways quite impossible in nature."[4]

Similar sentiments were expressed in *Genetically Engineered Food: A Self-Defense Guide for Consumers* by Ronnie Cummins, national director of the Organic Consumers Association, and Ben Lilliston, a writer on farming and the environment and communications coordinator for the Institute for Agriculture and Trade Policy in Minneapolis. "Genetic engineering ... is a revolutionary new technology still in the early experimental stages of development. It enables molecular biologist to permanently alter the essential characteristics or genetic codes of living organisms. This technology has the awesome power to break down fundamental genetic barriers—not only between species but between humans, animals, and plants. . . . For the first time in history, the scientists and corporations using the technology have become, in effect, the architects, builders, and 'owners' of life."[5]

Introducing the genes of one type of food into another, thereby changing the genetic structure of an organism, gives the second plant or animal beneficial characteristics, such as resistance to disease, improved nutritional value, and better growth. These modifications enable foods to grow faster, stronger, or bigger, all while using far less pesticide. A 2000 article in *JAMA: The Journal of the American Medical Association* notes that, "The acreage devoted to herbicide-resistant crops has been expanding because planting them reduces the need to plow more ground, decreases the amount of herbicidal chemicals needed, produces higher yields, and can deliver a higher grade of grain and other products."[6]

Cross-breeding has been around for a long time. Many common fruits are a result of hybridization. Yet according to the International Food Information Council, traditional cross-breeding often requires a good deal of time. "It is necessary to breed several generations in order to not only obtain the desired trait, but also remove numerous unwanted traits."[7]

Biotechnology, on the other hand, adds a whole new dimension to selective breeding. Researchers are able to add one or a few desirable genes to create crops with specific beneficial traits. "Gene technology not only provides the potential to select the exact characteristics desired, but it also enables us to transfer genes for desired traits more precisely."[8]

For example, several years ago, when Craig Nessler was professor and head of the Department of Plant Pathology, Physiology, and Weed Science at Virginia Tech University (now Virginia Polytechnic Institute and State University), he inserted genes from rats into lettuce seeds. That produced leafy greens with much higher amounts of vitamin C. In fact, a 2001 article in *Genomics & Genetics Weekly* states that "he increased the level of vitamin C in lettuce by 700%."[9] Why did Nessler use rats? "The gene was readily available and rodents are natural producers of vitamin C."[10] (Unlike rats, humans are unable to make their own vitamin C. That is why the sailors who were traveling to the "New World" developed scurvy, while the rats on board thrived.) Previously, such science would have been unthinkable.

The International Food Information Council contends that biotech crops enable farmers to use less pesticide and gasoline. "Biotech crops have reduced pesticide applications by 379 million pounds—an amount that could fill a 15-mile train of railcars." Because biotech crops are better at controlling weeds, farmers reduce the amount of time that they need to till the soil with their tractors. "This change in procedure saved 464 million gallons of diesel fuel and decreased greenhouse gas emissions (carbon dioxide) by 22 billion pounds."[11]

In addition, a 2003 article in *Environmental Health Perspectives* notes other potential benefits that biotech crops may have. "Plants may also be developed in which toxin content is downgraded, immunizing proteins are expressed, fat/protein ratio is altered, palatability is increased, and appearance is more appealing.... Crops may be developed that naturally express vitamins or that are deficient in specific allergens...."[12]

It is almost impossible for the average consumer to know whether there are GMOs in his or her food. Playing on consumers' fears of the unknown, some innovative marketers include "No GMOs" notations on their labels. Yet the vast majority of products do not indicate whether they are composed of any genetically altered ingredients. The legal authority for food labeling rests with the U.S. Food and Drug Administration. The agency requires GMOs be labeled only if they differ significantly from their conventional counterparts, such as containing a potential allergen.[13]

Currently Commercialized GM Crops in the US

Soy (89%), Cotton (83%), Canola (75%), Corn (60%), Hawaiian papaya (more than 50%), Alfalfa, Zucchini, and Yellow Squash (small amount), Tobacco (Quest brand)

Some Foods That May Contain GM Ingredients

Infant formula, salad dressing, bread, cereal, hamburgers and hotdogs, margarine, mayonnaise, crackers, cookies, chocolate, candy, fried food, chips, veggie burgers, meat substitutes, ice cream, frozen yogurt, tofu, tamari, soy sauce, soy cheese, tomato sauce, protein powder, baking powder, alcohol, vanilla, powdered sugar, peanut butter, enriched flour, and pasta. Non-food items include cosmetics, soaps, detergents, shampoo, and bubble bath.[14]

SUPPORTERS AND OPPONENTS OF GMOS

Should consumers feel comfortable eating genetically altered food? The controversy surrounding GMOs, or Frankenfoods, as they are called by those who oppose them, is filled with heated discussion. In general, the federal government, big business, and many researchers and numerous well-respected publications maintain that genetically altered food is perfectly safe. They contend that GMOs offer the potential to feed healthier food to far larger numbers of people. That is of particular significance, they say, when considering the vast amounts of food needed to feed the populations of developing countries. And the need is staggering. According to the Union of Concerned Scientists, the world presently contains 700 million people who are "chronically undernourished." In the future, that statistics will only worsen. "Over the next 20 years, the world's population will probably double. The global food supply would need to double just to stay even, but to triple for the larger population to be fed adequately."[15]

But the Union of Concerned Scientists, as well as sizeable numbers of esteemed researchers, consumers, and environmental groups, does not believe that GMOs are the solution to world hunger. They worry that there may be health risks associated with eating GMOs for extended periods of time, and they are also concerned about the environmental impact. In Europe, particularly Great Britain, large numbers of people have supported a ban on GMOs. Grocery stores are refusing to carry foods containing GMOs. Other countries are following Britain's lead.

The most serious GMO controversy has centered on food labeling. Usually, opponents of GMOs favor labeling. They want to know which foods have been changed and believe that shoppers, when presented with such information on the label, would shy away from them. But some people who support GMOs also want labeling. They believe that such labeling would help consumers accept these products.

GMO HISTORY

Genetic engineering food research began in the 1980s. In 1990 the enzyme chymosin was the first genetically engineered food to receive the approval of the FDA. More than half of the hard cheese currently sold in the United States is made with chymosin produced by genetically engineered fungi. The rest is made with chymosin obtained from rennet, an enzyme from the stomachs of slaughtered calves. The genetically engineered product is purer and easier to obtain.

Two years later, in 1992, the FDA approved the first genetically engineered whole food—the Calgene Flavr Savr tomato, which became available for sale in 1994. Because of a change to a single gene, the Calgene Flavr Savr tomato ripened without getting soft. However, the tomato encountered a number of problems, such as an inability to tolerate shipping. *Genetically Engineered Food: Changing the Nature of Nature* notes that "the company experienced problems when they tried to harvest and transport their soft, ripe tomatoes in the same rough fashion used for most tomatoes, which are picked and shipped green."[16]

Nevertheless, genetic engineering moved forward. By 1996 genetically engineered seeds for corn and soybeans were available. These were followed by seeds for potatoes, canola, and cotton. *Your Right to Know*, which was published in 2007, states that "an estimated 87% of U.S. soy, 52% of U.S. corn, 55% of U.S. canola, and 79% of U.S. cotton are genetically engineered."[17]

REGULATION OF GMOS

The FDA regulates GMOs as it does any other food. If a new product contains food items that are already considered safe, the manufacturer does not need to obtain special permission to sell the item. So, for example, if a genetically engineered fish contained a gene from another type of fish, then it would not require any FDA approval. Approval would only be required if a new food contained an additive that is unknown and therefore not regarded as safe.

In 1992 the FDA determined that there would be exceptions to this rule. If a new food contained ingredients that were likely to trigger allergic reactions in allergic individuals or if the manufacturing process dramatically altered the nutritional content, a label would be required. Unfortunately, this is not as clear-cut as it may initially appear to be. Foods are constantly combined together to form new foods. Should everything be labeled? The government and sizeable numbers of people within the food industry say that such labeling would be confusing and expensive.

EarthSave International disagrees. To members of the organization, the genetic engineering of food introduces new proteins into the human and animal food chains. Humans are exposed to entirely new foods. "This was demonstrated in the mid-1990s when soybeans were outfitted with a gene from the Brazil nut. While the scientists had attempted to produce a healthier soybean, they ended up with a potentially deadly one. Blood tests from people allergic to Brazil nuts showed reactions to the beans. It was fortunately never put on the market." Moreover, there is no easy way to predict an allergic reaction. There are no tests to prove in advance that a genetically modified food is safe. "That's because people aren't usually allergic to a food until they have eaten it several times."[18]

It is true that the government has mandated the labeling of other products such as foods that are processed and those containing sulfites. Labels must note the source of hydrolyzed proteins; cigarette labels have a warning from the surgeon general. In *Genetically Engineered Food: Changing the Nature of Nature* Martin Teitel and Kimberly A. Wilson write, "Labels of other ingredients, qualities, quantities, or features don't seem to be a problem. A bag of candy purchased in an American market is almost covered with a wealth of label information ... Then there is a list of what is *not* in the candy, interesting to note since genfood manufacturers are especially resistant to labeling food GMO-free."[19]

ARGUMENTS IN FAVOR OF GMOS

Some people contend that the negative publicity that consumer groups generate about GMOs is most harmful to the world's most vulnerable people—the poor. They say that unlike residents of wealthier countries, large segments of the population of developing countries worry about dying from malnutrition and starvation. By using GMOs, farmers in developing countries may harvest more crops with less pesticide.

In "Opportunities for and Challenges to Plant Biotechnology Adoption in Developing Countries," Gary Toenniessen, of the Rockefeller Foundation, explains that 80 percent of the world's population lives in developing countries. "A recent analysis indicates that 127 million pre-school children suffer from vitamin-A deficiency, which can cause blindness and early death."[20] Moreover, iron deficiency among women of childbearing age is common. Those women are more likely to give birth to underweight children. "Roughly 24,000 people die each day from hunger and hunger-related causes, three-quarters of them children."[21]

Why are so many people living on so little food? According to Toenniessen, "the root cause is poverty." The people, who live in rural areas, make too little money from their small-scale farming. "They are often hindered by traditional farming methods, increasingly depleted soils, shrinking plots of land, scarce and unreliable water, inequitable land-distribution patterns, and inefficient or unfair markets."[22]

While Toenniessen acknowledges that biotechnology is unable to solve such deep-rooted poverty and hunger, he believes that it may be "a set of powerful new tools that can facilitate the production, multiplication, and distribution of improved crop varieties."[23]

U.S. Department of Agriculture researcher John W. Finley compares the current debates over GMOs to the early days of automobiles and airplanes. Once each of these means of transportation was involved in a fatal accident, they were condemned as unsafe. "The reaction has been the same to new technology throughout history. It is a basic one in our nature—fear of the unknown.... Well meaning and intelligent people are protesting any food that has originated from genetically altered seed stock, and the reasons are familiar: 'It's unnatural.' 'It's playing God.' 'It's dangerous.' In fact, what is being protested is fear of the unknown."[24] Finley said that researchers are just beginning to understand the potential benefits of this new technology—"one that could lead to nutritionally balanced foods, insect and drought resistant plants, super varieties that will grow in and feed developing nations."[25]

A 2003 article in *AgBioForum* maintains that genetically modified salmon has the potential to save lives. The authors believe that genetically modified salmon would be 15 percent less costly than regular salmon. As a result, more people would eat it, thereby consuming increased amounts of omega-3 fatty acids. That, in turn, would reduce the incidence of heart disease. The authors estimate that about 1,400 lives would be saved each year in the United States. "Regulators' focus on potential adverse health effects of GM foods, without regard to health benefits, does not provide an adequate basis for rational policy. Policies restricting the introduction of GM foods that offer lower-cost access to healthier foodstuffs may unintentionally curtail or postpone opportunities to improve public health."[26]

In *The Future of Food*, Brian J. Ford, an English scientist, writer, lecturer, and television host, says that a number of everyday farm animals and crops—such as pigs, cattle, wheat, oats, barley, and rye—are the result of human intervention. "Traditional farmers have been producing new animals and plants by cross-breeding for ten thousand years." While genetic engineering "offers a more radical way of manipulating characteristics," it is fast becoming part of daily life. "Genetic modification is inevitable. Like electric power, road transport, or computers, it is a fact of the future and the public will gain little by campaigning to ban this potentially rewarding technology. Properly applied, it could offer us so much."[27]

All the same, Ford does not believe that the public should simply accept whatever the bioengineering companies do. Rather, he calls for a careful monitoring of the industry and the introduction of safeguards. "This is a huge new industry, and it will have pronounced effects on us all.... We will need to control it."[28] Ford suggests the following controls:

- Approval for new experiments should always be sought from a regulatory authority well versed in the subject.
- None of the members of such a committee should be in a position to benefit commercially from approval.
- No genes conferring problematical properties (e.g., antibiotic resistance) shall be used, whether as markers or otherwise, outside enclosed laboratories.
- Agents capable of transfer to wild plants, like pollen-carrying genes conferring resistance, shall not be liberated into the environment.
- The public shall be consulted about the siting and the benefits of experiments.
- All GMO products should be properly labeled and the source declared.
- Records of possible unwanted side effects should be meticulously maintained. All such events should be investigated by an organization unconnected with the source of the product.[29]

ARGUMENTS AGAINST GMOS

The controversy shows no sign of diminishing, and GMO opponents present some compelling arguments. They note that genetic engineering destroys the basic, elemental barriers between species. Unlike cross-breeding, which can only occur with life forms that are closely related, when genes from different species are combined, genetic codes are altered. Completely new organisms are created. This has the potential to compromise human health and well-being, animal welfare, and the environment. A 2006 article in *Environmental Nutrition* notes that "the chief concern is that genes from bioengineered plants or animals might inadvertently mix with natural genes, forever altering the planet's ecosystem in ways that are impossible to predict."[30]

The Council for Responsible Genetics notes that, "genetic engineering may cause unintended side effects that make foods hazardous for human consumption. Unpredictable gene expression may result in the unanticipated toxic effects or allergies. We have indisputable evidence that genetically engineered food may produce serious, even fatal, allergic reactions."[31]

The Council is also worried about seeds that have been engineered to be more herbicide tolerant. They are able to withstand more frequent applications of chemical herbicides. "The long-term health consequences of these synthetic chemicals are unknown, but many of the chemicals are known to cause birth defects or cancer in laboratory animals and are toxic to fish."[32]

And what about world hunger? Surely, GMOs could be part of the solution.The Council disagrees. The hundreds of millions of people who are hungry do not have access to food. "They lack the money to buy it, and they lack the land to grow it." In addition, "private biotech corporations prevent small farmers from reusing their seeds, a traditional practice that provides food security for 1.4 billion people."[33]

An article published in 2004 in *Women's Health Letter* underscores the very real concern of allergic reactions. The article describes how a woman named Grace Booth had trouble breathing after eating corn tortillas in a restaurant. The corn tortillas had been made with StarLink corn, which was genetically modified with a gene from an insecticide. StarLink never received approval for human consumption, and it was removed from the market. Yet in 2003 "a U.S. testing program found more than one percent of all corn samples by farmers contained traces of StarLink."[34]

A 2002 article in *Environmental Health Perspectives* notes that in the United States about seven million people have documented food allergies. "The only treatment for food allergies is dietary avoidance, which depends upon being able to identify the source of exposure and treat reactions should they occur." However, because no GMO labeling is required, "it is impossible to know whether the produce one buys at the supermarket contains possible allergenic transgenic proteins."[35]

Even some animals have been found to refuse to eat genetically modified foods. For example, "a farmer in the Netherlands put two piles of corn in his mouse-infested barn. One was genetically engineered. The other wasn't. The mice ate every bit of the non-GM rice, but didn't touch the GM pile." In another instance, "a soybean farmer in Illinois had to fight off soybean-loving geese every year until he planted a small area with GM soybeans. The geese ate every bit of the non-GM soybeans and left the altered ones alone." And farmers in the Midwest watched cows walk past fields of genetically altered corn and eat non-GM corn right down to the ground, cornstalk and all."[36]

Another serious problem is raised by an article published in 2006 in the environmental magazine *E.* "Currently, all safety testing of genetically modified foods is done by the same companies that do the research, development and selling of bioengineered plants." Critics have faulted the FDA for this practice, and they have asked for the FDA to conduct its own testing. But "the FDA sees this system as adequate, and less expensive than its government-sponsored alternative."[37]

A 2006 article in *Environmental Nutrition* offers a number of suggestions for avoiding genetically modified foods. First, eat as much organic food as possible. By definition, organic foods may not be genetically modified. Patronize stores that do not carry GMOs such as Whole Foods, Wild Oats, and Trader Joe's. Scan labels for possible GM ingredients such as soy oil, soy sauce, corn oil, corn syrup, cornstarch, lecithin, cottonseed oil, and canola oil. Also, check foods on the comprehensive "The True Food Shopping List" at the Greenpeace USA website (http://www.greenpeace.org).[38]

CONCLUSION

The controversy surrounding genetically modified foods shows no signs of diminishing. Each year, increasing numbers of farmers grow more and more acres of genetically modified foods. These crops are able to enhance yields, protect against stressors, decrease the use of pesticides and herbicides, and extend shelf life. But, are these benefits taking a toll on the health and well-being of consumers and the environment? For now, there is no definitive answer to that question.

NOTES

1. GEO-PIE Cooperative Extension Program, Cornell University website, http://geo-pie.cornell.edu.

2. GEO-PIE Cooperative Extension Program, Cornell University website.

3. International Service for the Acquisition of Agri-Biotech Applications website, http://www.isaaa.org.

4. Martin Teitel and Kimberly A. Wilson, *Genetically Engineered Food: Changing the Nature of Nature* (Rochester, Vermont: Park Street Press, 2001) 1–2.

5. Ronnie Cummins and Ben Lilliston, *Genetically Engineered Food: A Self-Defense Guide for Consumers* (New York: Marlowe& Company, 2004) 17.

6. Charles Marwick, Charles, "Genetically Modified Crops Feed Ongoing Controversy," *JAMA: The Journal of the American Medical Association* (January 12, 2000) 283: 188–90.

7. International Food Information Council website, http://www.ific.org.

8. International Food Information Council website.

9. "Genes Increase Vitamin C in Plants." *Genomics & Genetics Weekly* (August 24, 2001) 11.

10. "Genes Increase Vitamin C in Plants."

11. International Food Information Council website.

12. Dean D. Metcalfe, "Introduction: What Are the Issues in Addressing the Allergenic Potential of Genetically Modified Foods?" *Environmental Health Perspectives* (June 15, 2003) 111: 1110–13.

13. U. S. Food and Drug Administration website, http://www.fda.gov.

14. Jeffrey M. Smith, *Genetic Roulette: The Documented Health Risks of Genetically Engineered Foods* (Fairfield, Iowa: Yes! Books, 2007) 258.

15. Union of Concerned Scientists website, http://www.ucsusa.org.

16. Martin Teiltel and Kimberly A. Wilson, *Genetically Engineered Food: Changing the Nature of Nature*, 23.

17. Andrew Kimbrell, *Your Right to Know* (San Rafael, California: Earth Aware Editions, 2007).

18. EarthSave International website, http://www.earthsave.org.

19. Martin Teitel and Kimberly A. Wilson, *Genetically Engineered Food: Changing the Nature of Nature*, 63.

20. Gary Toenniessen, "Opportunities for and Challenges to Plant Biotechnology Adoption in Developing Countries," The Rockefeller Foundation website, http://www.rockfound.org, 245.

21. Gary Toenniessen, "Opportunities for and Challenges to Plant Biotechnology Adoption in Developing Countries," 245.

22. Gary Toenniessen, "Opportunities for and Challenges to Plant Biotechnology Adoption in Developing Countries," 246.

23. Gary Toenniessen, "Opportunities for and Challenges to Plant Biotechnology Adoption in Developing Countries," 260.

24. John W. Finley, "Genetically Modified Foods: Agriculture's Bright Future or Dark Nightmare?" U.S. Department of Agriculture's website, http://www.usda.gov.

25. John W. Finley, "Genetically Modified Foods: Agriculture's Bright Future or Dark Nightmare?"

26. Randall Lutter and Katherine Tucker, "Unacknowledged Health Benefits of Genetically Modified Food: Salmon and Heart disease Deaths," *AgBioForum* (January 31, 2003) 5: 59–64.

27. Brian J. Ford, *The Future of Food* (New York: Thames and Hudson, 2000) 64–5.

28. Brian J. Ford, *The Future of Food*, 66.

29. Brian J. Ford, *The Future of Food*, 78.

30. "Genetically Modified Foods: The Uninvited Guests at Your Dinner Table," *Environmental Nutrition* (January 2006) 29(1): 3.

31. Council for Responsible Genetics website, http://www.gene-watch.org.

32. Council for Responsible Genetics website.

33. Council for Responsible Genetics website.

34. "Five Ways Genetically Modified Foods Threaten Your Health and What You Can Eat Instead," *Women's Health Letter* (April 2004) 10: 1–4.

35. Mary Eubanks, "Allergies a la Carte: Is there a Problem with Genetically Modified Foods?" *Environmental Health Perspectives* (March 2002) 110: A130–A131.

36. "Five Ways Genetically Modified Foods Threaten Your Health and What You Can Eat Instead," 1–4.

37. Starre Vartan, "Ah-tchoo! Do Genetically Modified Foods Cause Allergies?" *E* (November—December 2006) 17: 40–1.

38. "Genetically Modified Foods: The Uninvited Guests at Your Dinner Table," *Environmental Nutrition* (January 2006) 29: 3.

REFERENCES AND RESOURCES

Books

Cummins, Ronnie and Ben Lilliston. *Genetically Engineered Food: A Self-Defense Guide for Consumers.* New York: Marlowe & Company, 2004.

Kimbrell, Andrew. *Your Right to Know.* San Rafael, California: Earth Aware Editions, 2007.

Smith, Jeffrey M. *Genetic Roulette: The Documented Health Risks of Genetically Engineered Foods.* Fairfield, Iowa: Yes! Books, 2007.

Teitel, Martin and Kimberly A Wilson. *Genetically Engineered Food: Changing the Nature of Nature.* Rochester, Vermont: Park Street Press, 2001.

Magazines, Journals, and Newspapers

Eubanks, Mary. "Allergies a la Carte: Is There a Problem with Genetically Modified Foods?" *Environmental Health Perspectives* (March 2002) 110: A130–A131.

"Five Ways Genetically Modified Foods Threaten Your Health and What You Can Eat Instead." *Women's Health Letter* (April 2004) 10: 1–4.

Ford, Brian J. *The Future of Food.* New York: Thames and Hudson, 2000.

"Genes Increase Vitamin C in Plants." *Genomics & Genetics Weekly* (August 24, 2001) 11.

"Genetically Modified Foods: The Uninvited Guests at Your Dinner Table." *Environmental Nutrition* (January 2006) 2: 3.

"Genetically Modified Foods: The Uninvited Guests at Your Dinner Table." *Environmental Nutrition* (January 2006) 29: 3.

Kennedy, Rozella. "Genetically Engineered Foods: Too Many Unknowns. *Mothering* (March—April 2000) 40.

Lutter, Randall and Katherine Tucker. "Unacknowledged Health Benefits of Genetically Modified Foods: Salmon and Heart Disease Deaths." *AgBioForum* (January 31, 2003) 5: 59–64.

Marwick, Charles. "Genetically Modified Crops Feed Ongoing Controversy." *JAMA: The Journal of the American Medical Association* (January 12, 2000) 283: 188–90.

Metcalfe, Dean D. "Introduction: What Are the Issues in Addressing the Allergenic Potential of Genetically Modified Foods?" *Environmental Health Perspectives* (June 15, 2003) 111: 1110–13.

Vartan, Starre. "Ah-tchoo! Do Genetically Modified Foods Cause Allergies?" *E* (November—December 2006) 17: 40–1.

Websites

BioScience Productions
http://www.actionbioscience.org

Center for Food Safety
http://www.centerforfoodsafety.org

Cooperative Extension Program, Cornell University
http://geo-pie.cornell.edu

Council for Responsible Genetics
http://www.gene-watch.org

Greenpeace USA
http://www.greenpeace.org

EarthSave International
http://earthsave.org

International Food Information Council
http://www.ific.org

International Service for the Acquisition of Agri-Biotech Applications
http://www.isaaa.org

The Rockefeller Foundation
http://www.rockfound.org

Union of Concerned Scientists
http://www.ucsusa.org

U. S. Department of Agriculture
http://www.usda.gov

U.S. Food and Drug Administration
http://www.fda.gov

Chapter 9

Hidden Ingredients in Food

Sometimes, it is a challenge to determine what ingredients are in certain foods. Foods may contain hidden ingredients that can threaten the health and well-being of certain people. By design or by accident, foods may have ingredients not listed on the label. The Food and Drug Administration (FDA) allows trace amounts of natural products to be omitted from the label. It also takes no exception to the failure of manufacturers to mention the small amounts of insects, mold, and rodent filth may make their way into foods during processing. For example, the FDA permits cochineal, an insect, to be used as red coloring. After years of not being required to list it on labels, it now must be noted. But labels need not state that it is derived from insects.[1] A 2007 article in *This Magazine* says that Minute Maid Pink Grapefruits juice is made with cochineal.[2]

NATURAL FLAVORINGS

The term "natural flavorings" sounds so healthful. However, Title 21, Section 101, Part 22 of the Code of Federal Regulations defines natural flavorings as follows: "The term natural flavor or natural flavoring means the essential oil, oleoresin, essence or extractive, protein hydrolysate, distillate, or any product of roasting, heating or enzymolysis, which contains the flavoring constituents derived from a spice, fruit or fruit juice, vegetable or vegetable juice, edible yeast, herb, bark, bud, root, leaf or similar plant material, meat, seafood, poultry, eggs, dairy products, or fermentation products thereof, whose significant function in food is flavoring rather than nutritional."[3] So what is natural flavoring? What does the definition mean? The Vegetarian Resource Group notes, "Natural flavors can be pretty much anything approved for use in food."[4] As a result, unless a company specifically lists the source of its natural ingredients on the label, the consumer is left without a clue.

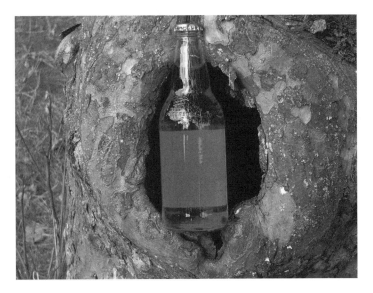

The red color of this soda may be due to cochineal, an insect. (Courtesy of Mark A. Goldstein)

A few, primarily smaller companies, do list sources, but the vast majority do not. Most consumers probably do not realize the types of hidden ingredients that may be the "natural flavorings" in their food.

In the bestselling *Fast Food Nation*, which has been reprinted many times since it was first released in 2001, Eric Schlosser noted that a number of food products obtain their flavors from unexpected sources. For example, the BK Broiler Chicken Breast Patty sold at Burger King has "natural smoke flavor." Schlosser says that the Red Arrow Products Company "manufactures natural smoke flavor by charring sawdust and capturing the aroma chemicals released into the air. The smoke is captured in water and then bottled, so that other companies can sell food which seems to have been cooked over a fire."[5]

The FDA contends that "it is economically impractical to grow, harvest, or process raw products that are totally free of non-hazardous, naturally occurring, unavoidable defects." However, the FDA does set limits, and it is against the law for manufacturers to exceed them. The limits are listed in a report entitled *The Food Defect Actions Levels*, and it may be found on the website of the U. S. Food and Drug Administration. (http://vm.cfsan.fda.gov/~dms/dalbook.html). The FDA maintains that manufacturers do not simply attempt to remain slightly below the permissible level. "The defect levels do not represent an average of the defects that occur in any of the products—the averages are actually much lower. The levels represent limits at which FDA would regard the food product 'adulterated' and subject to enforcement action."[6]

By becoming a diligent reader of food labels, one may try to avoid foods with natural flavorings, especially those in which the natural flavorings are not identified. While this is difficult and time-consuming, it may work with products purchased at a store, but vigilant label reading is of little assistance with restaurant or take-out foods. It is of no help with processed foods that may contain FDA-permissible amounts of insects, mold, and rodent filth.

Would organic foods be less likely to be tainted? As noted in chapter 13, the term *organic* relates to the way in which the food is grown and produced, not the method in which it is processed. Like other foods, natural flavorings would be listed as an ingredient of processed organic food. As long as they remain within FDA limits, they may have the same contaminants.

AVOIDING HIDDEN INGREDIENTS

As a result of concerns about hidden ingredients, a number of Jewish and non-Jewish people are eating more kosher products. According to Rabbi Eliezer Eidlitz, who maintains the website KosherQuest, about one-third of the products sold in supermarkets are certified kosher, and the interest in kosher foods continues to grow rapidly. Why? Although for some it is part of their religious practice and/or personal convictions, "most of the interest comes from people who feel that the kosher certification is their best guarantee that the products and ... ingredients are being watched carefully and properly."[7] There are no hidden ingredients in kosher foods. All ingredients are noted on the label. Moreover, the certifying agency tracks each ingredient to its ultimate source. "In the U. S. alone, there appear to be at least five million people who buy products based on their being kosher."[8]

More people are reducing their intake of processed foods. A newly washed tomato is exactly that—a tomato. However, the FDA allows canned tomatoes to have something more than tomatoes—"no more than 10 or more drosophila fly eggs per 500 grams or 5 or more drosophila fly eggs and 1 or more maggots per 500 grams or 2 or more maggots per 500 grams." In addition, 500 grams of berries may have 4 larvae or 10 whole insects.[9]

Although some people will be shocked to learn what may be in their food, for other people—those with food allergies and intolerances—such unknown ingredients may trigger significant negative reactions. For them, even small amounts of certain foods hidden in other foods may make them ill. A reaction from a food allergy may actually kill. Allergic reactions are not uncommon occurrences. According to The Food Allergy & Anaphylaxis Network, about 11 million Americans suffer from food allergy. Of these, 6.5 are allergic to seafood and 3 million are allergic to peanuts or tree nuts. Every year, about 150–200 Americans die from an allergic reaction to foods.[10]

Those who are allergic have no choice but to avoid the allergen. They should begin by reading ingredient labels, or they may attempt to contact the manufacturer. Unless a person with food allergies is able to determine that the food is safe, the food should not be consumed.

But that is sometimes easier said than done. Hoping to study the situation, the FDA formed a partnership with the Minnesota Department of Agriculture and the Wisconsin Department of Agriculture. They decided to begin a two-year investigation of the eight foods that cause 90 percent of the severe life-threatening reactions: peanuts, eggs, milk and milk products, wheat, tree nuts, soy, fish, and shellfish. In total, there were eighty-five companies.

For those with food allergies, the findings were disturbing. A number of bakers cross-contaminated foods because they used the same utensils for different mixes or reused baking sheets without washing them. Parchment papers were sometimes used as many as ten times before being replaced. One conveyor belt that coated candies in chocolate was cleaned only once a year.[11]

A 2006 article in *The Food Institute Report* says that foods may become cross-contaminated with a major food allergen during almost any step in the manufacturing process. The following are some of means of cross-contamination:

- Allergens in raw ingredients or processing aids
- Improper use of rework where rework product contains allergens
- Allergen carryover from use of shared equipment
- Use of clean-in-place fluid to clean shared equipment
- Methods of growing and harvesting crops
- Shared storage, transportation, or production equipment[12]

In *Peanut Butter, Milk, and Other Deadly Threats*, which was published in 2006, Sherri Mabry Gordon discusses cross-contamination and how easily it may occur. "An example may be a peanut butter cookie made on the same machine as a sugar cookie. Even though the machine may be thoroughly cleaned, the sugar cookie may contain traces of peanut."[13] People with allergies to milk are also at risk when cooking oil is reused, as might occur when French fries are cooked in the same oil as cheese sticks. The same is true when utensils, pots and pans, and kitchen equipment are used for several tasks before they are washed. "An example would be using a spatula to pick up a brownie with walnuts and then reusing that same spatula to pick up a piece of cornbread. The cornbread might contain traces of walnuts."[14] Steam or splattering may unintentionally combine foods. "An example would be boiling lobster next to a pot of soup. The splatter and/or steam from the lobster could get into the soup. As a result, the soup may contain traces of shellfish."[15]

Cross-contamination may occur in many places. Lisa Cipriano Collins, who has a son with severe peanut and tree nut allergies, observed in *Caring for Your Child with Severe Food Allergies*, which was published in 2000: "You need to imagine the production of foods and consider the possibility that cross-contamination can occur in raw material containers, processing machinery, packaging machinery, and display cases."[16] It is important to realize that chefs and their assistants do not necessarily understand that the foods causing allergic reactions must have no contact with the food that will be eaten by the allergic patron. It is not appropriate to simply take away the nuts from a salad that has been returned. Someone who is sensitive to nuts may still have a reaction, even after the nuts have been removed. A new nutless salad must be prepared. An individual who is sensitive to wheat cannot eat wheatless pancakes that have been made on the same griddle as wheat-based pancakes.

In *The Parent's Guide to Food Allergies*, which was published in 2001, Marianne S. Barber, Maryanne Bartoszek, and Elinor Greenberg note that cross-contamination with ice cream containing nuts is a risk in ice cream parlors. At a deli counter, a child who is highly allergic to dairy is at risk if ham or turkey has been sliced with a blade just used for cheese. (An establishment that adheres strictly to kosher rules will have separate slicers for meats and cheeses.) Similarly, at a salad bar, tongs may have just held shredded cheese or other salad ingredients containing milk products. "When eating in restaurants, it's best to bring a safe meal with you or order the simplest meal possible: plain grilled meat or chicken, baked potato, and salad or vegetable.... Anytime you are dealing with more than one ingredient, keep your antennae up. If your child loves hamburgers, you'll have to find out if the patties are 100 percent beef—there could be soy, wheat, even egg or other fillers hiding in there. If the allergy is to milk, egg, soy, wheat, peanuts or nuts, bring your own dessert."[17]

In *The Complete Peanut Allergy Handbook*, which was published in 2005, Scott H. Sicherer and Terry Malloy depict a number of actual instances of hidden peanuts in foods obtained outside the home. Some of these are as follows:

- A piecrust has peanut embedded in it, so you couldn't actually see the nuts.
- An ice cream cone had a face on it made from small chocolate-covered candies, and one of them had peanut on it. The family asked if the candies contained peanut, and the salesperson said, 'Oh no, those are just chocolate,' but they turned out to be chocolate-covered peanut candies.
- Egg roll was sealed with peanut butter, or, in another situation, had peanut flour in it.

- A garnish in a salad had finely chopped peanuts.
- A jelly sandwich, just like the kind that can be made in the home, was contaminated with peanut, because the jelly had previously been used for a peanut butter and jelly sandwich.[18]

In *The Peanut Allergy Answer Book*, which was published in 2006, Michael C. Young notes that because of its ability to enhance flavor and texture, peanut butter is added to a host of different cooked foods. "Peanut butter is often used as a shortening or oil in recipes for many types of gravy. It can give a smoother texture to sauces. It is also used as a thickener for many recipes. Peanut butter has adhesive properties that allow it to be used to 'glue down' the ends of eggs rolls to keep them from coming apart." Peanuts, peanut oil, and peanut butter are included in a variety of international foods such as Chinese, Japanese, Indian, Ethiopian, Mexican, African, Vietnamese, and Thai. "Sauces and toppings can have finely crushed peanuts mixed in without any visible sign of them.... Peanut flour is used in certain brands of frozen dinners. Slivered almonds found on some baked good may actually be made from raw peanuts because they are much cheaper."[19]

Lisa Cipriano Collins describes one case of an allergic reaction that was the basis for a lawsuit against a large restaurant chain. A woman who was allergic to nuts asked the waitress at the restaurant to list the ingredients of the pesto sauce. Because nuts were not on the list, she ordered it. When the dish was brought to the table, she asked the waitress directly if the sauce had nuts in it. The waitress allegedly said that no nuts were in the sauce, but it contained both pine nuts and walnuts. The woman went into anaphylactic shock and later died.[20]

Cross-contamination may easily occur in the grocery store. Bulk-food bins are at high risk for cross-contamination from other foods, especially if they are not thoroughly cleaned between uses. Juices from foods may leak onto other foods in the grocery cart. Any such food should be tightly wrapped in a plastic bag before it is placed in the cart.

There is similar concern about the contamination of pareve foods. Although the exact origin of the word is unknown, pareve essentially means that the food lies between the extremes of meat and dairy. Pareve foods, which contain a label with a U in a circle or the word *pareve*, contain no meat or dairy derivatives. They have not been cooked or mixed with any meat or dairy foods and may be eaten with both meat and milk foods. Eggs, fish, fruit, vegetables, grains, and juices in their unprocessed state are common pareve foods. Other pareve foods include pasta, soft drinks, coffee, tea, and many types of candy and snacks. During processing, however, the pareve designation may be rendered meaningless. Pareve foods may lose their pareve status if they are processed on equipment that was used to process dairy products. According to Rabbi Simcha Smolensky, of the Chicago Rabbinical Council, people with allergies should not rely on this designation. "With the complexities of food processing, it is not hard to imagine that in a plant that makes both pareve and dairy items, a very small quantity of a dairy ingredient could find its way into an otherwise pareve product."[21]

Though they may have different reasons for discomfort, vegetarians, who do not eat animal foods but do eat dairy products, and vegans, who eliminate animal and dairy products, worry about hidden ingredients in their foods. Vegetarians and vegans may have various motivations for choosing their diets—animals rights and/or personal health—but they do not want to eat a seemingly vegan food, such as guacamole, that contains food from an animal, such as gelatin, or hash browns that have been fried in the same oil as meat or seafood products. The website of The Vegetarian Resource Group (http://www.vrg.org) contains a listing of vegetarian-, vegan-, and/or vegetarian-friendly restaurants in the United States. Furthermore, the North American Vegetarian Society warns of inaccurate labeling. Manufacturers may contend that their products contain no animal ingredients when, in fact, they have foods such as honey, whey, casein, and bone rennet, all of which come from animals.[22]

In *Raising Vegetarian Children*, which was published in 2002, Joanne Stepaniak and Vesanto Melina mention other "more common but often overlooked animal-derived ingredients." One example is oleic acid. Used to flavor or bind ingredients, oleic acid is derived from the fat of pigs or cows. Another example is gelatin, which is used to thicken or gel "puddings, yogurt, marshmallows, sour cream, frozen desserts, cheese spreads, and the capsules of pills and supplements." It is an animal protein obtained from cows or pigs. Still another example is royal jelly, a product produced by the glands of bees that is used "to fortify with B vitamins, minerals and amino acids." It is often found in nutritional supplements.[23]

In Eric Schlosser's *Fast Food Nation*, the author describes the French fries sold at McDonald's restaurants. The McDonald's Corporation has refused to disclose the source of the natural flavoring used in the fries. "However, in response to inquires from *Vegetarian Journal* ... McDonald's did acknowledge that its fries derive some of their characteristic flavor from 'animal products.'"[24]

A 2002 article in *Caterer & Hotelkeeper* notes that cheese products may be made with the milk-curdling agent rennet, which normally is obtained from the stomachs of calves that have yet to be weaned. "Mistakes are often made when a chef or manufacturer uses ingredients in which meat products are hidden."[25]

A 2001 article in *The New York Times* describes how some New York City chefs were adding hidden ingredients such as tripe, pork jowls, and pigs' feet and calling them "secret spices." So as not to offend "the squeamish, they follow a silent rule: if you can't see it on the plate, you don't have to mention it on the menu." Clearly, this is not possible with some menu items. "Menu editing works with ingredients that disappear in the dish or are served on the side, but not with foods that are the main part of a dish, like snails."[26]

Despite the many advances, there is a growing awareness that some ingredients are still not listed on food labels. A number of national organizations and countless Internet sites may provide information. Many fast food restaurants post lists of all their ingredients in their products. Whenever possible, these include the "hidden ones." Lists may also be obtained on the Internet. Certainly, in better restaurants, when a diner notifies a member of the wait staff of a food allergy or intolerance, the server will quickly provide information or check with the chef. Chefs and the members of their staff are becoming increasingly aware of the problem and adjusting their meals to suit the needs of their customers.

CONCLUSIONS

When eating away from home, people with food allergies must always be cautious. They should veer in the direction of eating plain foods with fewer ingredients. They should ask for food that has been kept separate and prepared in a carefully washed pan. They should support and patronize restaurants and stores that cater to their needs. Above all, they should continue to speak out, raise public awareness, and write letters to their congressional representatives asking for stricter food standards. If legislators believe that there is a strong constituency for these issues, they will respond with new laws and increased resources.

TOPICS FOR DISCUSSION

1. Before reading this chapter, did you realize what natural flavorings were? Has the chapter influenced how you feel about them? Why or why not?

2. Do you have any friends who have food allergies? Has your school made adequate provisions for them? List a few ways in which your school could make further improvements.

3. Pretend you are allergic to peanuts. Think of five ways you could reduce your chances of cross-contamination in a restaurant.

4. What are some of the ways that restaurant personnel may be better educated about the seriousness of food allergies? Devise a few strategies.

5. What should be the FDA's role regarding standards for food? Are the current standards sufficient? Why or why not?

NOTES

1. Center for Science in the Public Interest, email exchange, cspinews@cspinet.org.

2. Sarah Ferguson and Stacy Lee Kong, "Four Things That May Not Be As Good For You As You Think," *This Magazine* (March–April 2007) 40: 10.

3. U. S. Food and Drug Administration website, http://www.fda.gov.

4. The Vegetarian Resource Group website, http://www.vfg.org.

5. Eric Schlosser, *Fast Food Nation* (New York: Harper Perennial, 2005) 128.

6. U.S. Food and Drug Administration website.

7. KosherQuest website, http://kosherquest.org.

8. KosherQuest website.

9. U.S. Food and Drug Administration website.

10. The Food Allergy & Anaphylaxis Network website, www.foodallergy.org.

11. Greg Winter, "F.D.A. Survey Finds Faulty Listings of Possible Food Allergens," *New York Times* (April 3, 2001) Section C, page1 column 2.

12. "Food Allergen Report Summarized," *The Food Institute Report* (September 18, 2006) 39: 9.

13. Sherri Mabry Gordon, *Peanut Butter, Milk, and Other Deadly Threats* (Berkeley Heights, New Jersey: Enslow Publishers, Inc., 2006) 47–48.

14. Sherri Mabry Gordon, *Peanut Butter, Milk, and Other Deadly Threats*, 48.

15. Sherri Mabry Gordon, *Peanut Butter, Milk, and Other Deadly Threats*, 48.

16. Lisa Cipriano Collins, *Caring for Your Child with Severe Food Allergies* (New York: John Wiley and Sons, 2000) 31.

17. Marianne S. Barber, Maryanne Bartoszek Scott, and Elinor Greenberg, *The Parent's Guide to Food Allergies* (New York: Henry Holt and Company, 2001) 118–9.

18. Scott H. Sicherer and Terry Malloy, *The Complete Peanut Allergy Handbook* (New York: Berkeley Books, 2005) 203.

19. Michael C. Young, *The Peanut Allergy Answer Book* (Gloucester, Massachusetts: Fair Winds Press, 2006) 101.

20. Lisa Cipriano Collins, *Caring for Your Child with Severe Food Allergies*, 27.

21. Rabbi Simcha Smolensky, "Is Pareve Really Pareve?" Chicago Rabbinical Council website, http://www.crcweb.org.

22. North American Vegetarian Society website, http://navs-online.org.

23. Joanne Stepaniak and Vesanto Melina, *Raising Vegetarian Children*, (Chicago and other cities: Contemporary Books, 2002).

24. Eric Schlosser, *Fast Food Nation*, 128.

25. Bob Gledhill, "One Man's Meat," *Caterer & Hotelkeeper* (April 11, 2002) 54.

26. Melissa Clark, "Menus That Don't Tell the Whole Story," *The New York Times* (January 24, 2001) Section F, page 3, column 1.

REFERENCES AND RESOURCES

Books

Barber, Marianne S., Maryanne Bartoszek Scott, and Elinor Greenberg. *The Parent's Guide to Food Allergies*. New York: Henry Holt and Company, 2001.

Cipriano Collins, Lisa. *Caring for Your Child with Severe Food Allergies*. New York: John Wiley and Sons, 2000.

Mabry Gordon, Sherri. *Peanut Butter, Milk, and Other Deadly Threats*. Berkeley Heights, New Jersey: Enslow Publishers, Inc., 2006.

Schlosser, Eric. *Fast Food Nation*. New York: Harper Perennial, 2005.

Sicherer, Scott H. and Terry Malloy. *The Complete Peanut Allergy Handbook*. New York: Berkeley Books, 2005.

Stepaniak, Joanne and Vesanto Melina. *Raising Vegetarian Children*. Chicago and other cities: Contemporary Books, 2002.
Young, Michael C. *The Peanut Allergy Book*. Gloucester, Massachusetts: Fair Winds Press, 2006.

Magazines, Journals, and Newspapers

Clark, Melissa. "Menus That Don't Tell the Whole Story." *The New York Times* (January 24, 2001) Section F, page 3, column 1.
Ferguson, Sarah and Stacy Lee Kong. "Four Things That May Not Be As Good For You As You Think." *This Magazine* (March–April 2007) 40: 10.
"Food Allergen Report Summarized." *The Food Institute Report* (September 18, 2006) 39: 9.
Gledhill, Bob. "One Man's Meat." *Caterer & Hotelkeeper* (April 11, 2002) 54.
Winter, Greg. "F.D.A. Survey Finds Faulty Listings of Possible Food Allergens." *New York Times* (April 3, 2001) Section C, page 1, column 2.

Websites

Center for Science in the Public Interest
http://www.cspinet.org

Chicago Rabbinical Council
http://www.crcweb.org

KosherQuest
http://kosherquest.org

North American Vegetarian Society
http://navs-online.org

The Food Allergy & Anaphylaxis Network
www.foodallergy.org

The Vegetarian Resource Group
http://www.vrg.org

U. S. Food and Drug Administration
http://www.fda.gov

Chapter 10

Imported Food

No dog or cat lover can easily forget March 2007. That is when manufacturers began recalling over 100 brands of dog and cat food. Something in the food was causing the animals to develop kidney failure. Many dogs and cats died well before their time.

It did not take the Food and Drug Administration (FDA) long to determine that some pet food (in addition to feed for chickens, farmed fish, and pigs) had been contaminated with the two industrial chemicals melamine and cyanuric acid. A July 18, 2007 report presented to the U.S. Senate Commerce Committee noted that "these toxins were found in wheat gluten imported from China and used in many pet food and animal feed products manufactured in the U.S. Chinese wheat gluten producers are thought to have intentionally contaminated the product with melamine to give the appearance of increased protein content."[1]

Though tainted food from China seems to garner a good deal of media attention, food from other countries has also caused illness in the United States. In the fall of 2003 there was a large outbreak of hepatitis A in Pennsylvania, Georgia, Tennessee, and North Carolina. In Pennsylvania alone, hundreds of people were sickened. Of these, a few died. The outbreaks in Pennsylvania, Georgia, and Tennessee were traced to green onions grown in Mexico. The Food and Drug Administration was never able to locate the source of the outbreak in North Carolina. In all instances, the contaminated green onions were consumed in restaurants. Still, the FDA determined that four Mexican growers were involved in the outbreaks. Though there was no direct evidence of hepatitis A on the four farms, the extremely poor sanitary conditions, inadequate hand-washing facilities, and concerns over the health and welfare of workers presented ideal conditions for the development of the disease. Moreover, the quality of the water used in the field, packing sheds, and ice making

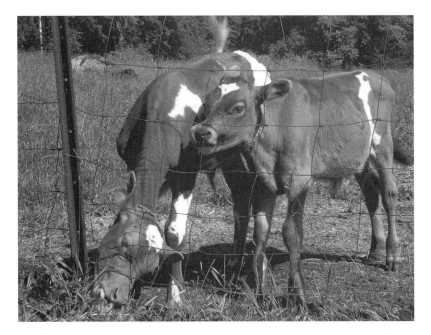

Beef raised in the U.S. is inspected. (Courtesy of Mark A. Goldstein)

was questionable. "There is rarely any physical evidence in a foodborne illness outbreak. By the time people begin to show symptoms of illness, the contaminated food has been consumed or discarded. In the case of hepatitis A, which has a long incubation period [10–50 days, average of 30 days], there is even less likelihood of existence of produce that can be tested for the presence of contamination."[2]

An article entitled "U.S. Food Safety: The Import Alarm Keeps Sounding," which was published in January 2008 by *U.S. News & World Report*, offers more information about the conditions found on these farms. Dirty shower water flowed directly onto the fields where the cantaloupes grew. Apparently, the water contained filthy diapers and soiled feminine hygiene products. "The growing fields were irrigated with water from a pond that was also a dumping ground for human sewage and animal manure. During processing, green onions typically passed through the hands of at least six workers ... and there was no evidence that the workers were allowed time off for illness."[3]

Similarly, between 2000 and 2002, there were three multistate Salmonella serotype Poona infections that came from eating cantaloupe from farms in Mexico. When the FDA representatives investigated the farms, they "found many possible sources of contamination, including sewage-contaminated irrigation water, processing (cleaning and cooling) with

Salmonella-contaminated water, poor hygienic practices of handlers, pests in packing facilities, and inadequate cleaning and sanitizing of equipment that came in contact with the cantaloupe."[4] Still another Salmonella outbreak from cantaloupes from a Honduran grower was reported early in 2008. People became ill in at least sixteen states and Canada.[5]

An article in the May 2007 issue of *The American Journal of Public Health* reported on an outbreak of lead poisoning in Monterey County, California. Researchers determined that one of the significant risk factors was eating food imported from the Zimatlan area of Oaxaca, Mexico. In particular, researchers found that "home-prepared dried grasshoppers (chapulines) sent from Oaxaca were found to contain significant amounts of lead."[6]

These are only some of the food-related illnesses that make the news. The previously cited 2008 *U. S. News & World Report* article noted, "Food safety experts stress that it's almost impossible to sort out whether the thousands of smaller food-linked disease outbreaks that occur each year in the United States are attributable to domestic or imported product. According to the U.S. Centers for Disease Control and Prevention, about 76 million cases of food-related illness are reported in the United States each year, including 5,000 deaths."[7]

Obviously, these outbreaks raise a number of questions. How much food does the United States actually import? Does it really represent a sizeable amount of what U.S. residents consume? How does tainted food make its way into the United States? Aren't there systems in place to protect people and animals?

An April 16, 2007, article, entitled "Imported Food Rarely Inspected," in the *Washington Post* noted that in a typical year "the average American eats about 260 pounds of imported food, including processed, ready-to-eat products, and single ingredients. Imports account for about 13 percent of the annual diet."[8] Meanwhile, the U.S. Department of Agriculture (USDA) estimates that for the 12 months ending in September 2007, the United States imported $70 billion in agricultural products. (That is about double the amount that was imported in 1997.) "About one-quarter of our fruit, both fresh and frozen, is imported. For tree nuts, it's about half. And, for fish and shellfish, more than two-thirds come from overseas." But only a little more than one percent of these foods is inspected by the FDA before they enter the country.[9] (This is down from 1.8 percent in 1997.[10]) People are often shocked when they learn that the figure is so low. Although the federal government allocates about $1.7 billion for food safety, most of that money goes to the USDA, which regulates about 20 percent of the food supply. On the other hand, the FDA, which regulates about 80 percent of the food supply, receives only about 24 percent of the total amount spent on food safety.[11]

In the United States today, there are approximately 300 ports of entry for food. But only about 90 of these have full-time inspectors. When food is rejected at one point, it is not uncommon for the ship to move on to another port where it may avoid inspection. This is a practice known as "port shopping."[12]

An October 15, 2007, article in *Supermarket News* states that the FDA has fewer than 650 food inspectors. "Stretched as thin as they are, these inspectors are often unable to visit the fields and food production facilities that the agency is responsible for more often than once every three to five years."[13] So while the amount of imported food keeps rising, the amount of food that is inspected keeps going down. The previously mentioned July 18, 2007, report to the U.S. Senate Commerce Committee notes that "to increase inspections of FDA-regulated imports to 10 percent (still a strikingly low figure) would require an additional 1600 full-time inspectors and at least $270 million. To double that figure to 20 percent import inspection would require 3200 full-time inspectors and $540 million."[14]

As a result, FDA inspectors focus on those foods that have a history of being at higher risk. These include fruits and vegetables as well as fish and shellfish. "Foods from countries or producers previously shown to be problematic are also flagged for a closer look."[15] So what do FDA inspectors search for? A February 27, 2007, article in *The Houston Chronicle* says that they "look for filth, decomposition, adulteration with pesticides and industrial chemicals and the illegal use of color or food additives.... Inspectors also look for sources of possible contamination, such as flies.... They're also told to look for open doors or damaged window screens that could allow the insects to flit back and forth between the product and, say, a toilet, floor drain or garbage can."[16]

Moreover, an April 23, 2007, MSNBC article reports that inspectors rarely if ever investigate product ingredients. So, for example, they would not have examined the content of the contaminated pet food. To examine ingredients, the inspectors would need access to laboratories. "Analyzing samples takes days and can irk importers who don't like the choice of holding their product or risking a costly recall if they go ahead with distribution."[17] In general, buyers and suppliers must conduct their own quality control. "If they don't do it, they run the risk of health problems that can devastate a brand and generate huge lawsuits."[18]

But none of this information explains why there is such a dramatic difference in the allocation of resources between the USDA and the FDA. The previously noted October 15, 2007, *Supermarket News* article offers at least a partial explanation. In the article, Chris Waldrop, director of the Food Policy Institute at the Consumer Federation of America, says that there is a sharp difference in the laws governing the USDA and the FDA. The USDA requires continuous inspection of every slaughterhouse in the United States. "As a result, there's a statutory mandate that these inspectors must be employed at the plants on a regular basis. The FDA doesn't have the same mandate. They do inspections, but they only get to some food processing facilities once every five years or so.... Once every five years is simply inadequate."[19]

It is hard to find people who truly believe that the current system provides sufficient protection for the American public. A poll conducted in September 2006 "found that only 30 percent of the 1,000 randomly selected participants had a great deal of confidence that the agency [FDA] could ensure the safety of their food."[20] During May 2007, testimony before Congress, David Kessler, a former FDA commissioner, said, "our food safety system is broken."[21]

In February 8, 2007, testimony before the Subcommittee on Agriculture, Rural Development, FDA, and Related Agencies, Committee on Appropriations of the House of Representatives, David M. Walker, the Comptroller General of the United States, said that because of the problems inherent in the current food-monitoring programs there is increased risk that unsafe food remains in the food supply and is consumed. "Specifically, USDA and FDA do not know how promptly and completely the recalling companies and their distributors and other customers are carrying out recalls, and neither agency is using its data systems to effectively track and manage its recall programs. For these and other reasons, most recalled food is not recovered and therefore may be consumed."[22] Moreover, although the FDA has the authority to penalize a company up to $100,000 for failing to recall a "defective biological product, such as a vaccine," it has no authority "to penalize a company that is slow to conduct a food recall."[23]

Acknowledging problems with the FDA, a number of nonprofit groups (e.g., the American Heart Association and the American Red Cross), consumer groups (e.g., Center for Science in the Public Interest and Consumer Federation of America), industry groups (e.g., Consumer Health Care Products Association and the Council for Responsible Nutrition), companies (e.g., AstraZeneca and Pfizer), and former government officials (Mark B. McClellan, Tommy G. Thompson, Donna E. Shalala, and Louis Sullivan) joined together to form Coalition for a Stronger FDA. A multiyear effort, the Coalition was created to ensure that the FDA has sufficient resources "to protect patients and consumers and maintain public confidence and trust in the FDA."[24]

The Coalition notes that the FDA regulates about 25 percent of all consumer spending. Yet "FDA funding has lagged behind appropriations for other public health agencies over the last two decades."[25] The Coalition provides the following examples:

- In 1986, FDA's budget was $416.7 million—or 97 percent of the CDC's $429.4 million budget and 8 percent of NIH's $5.1 billion budget.
- In 1996, FDA's budget was $865 million—or 39 percent of CDC's $2.2 billion budget and 8 percent of NIH's $10.2 billion budget.
- In 2006, FDA's budget was $1.5 billion—or 28 percent of CDC's $5.2 billion budget and 5 percent of NIH's $27.7 billion budget.[26]

How does the Coalition plan to increase FDA funding? It hopes to work to increase awareness among policymakers as well as educate the public. "We plan to build awareness of the current deficiencies and new challenges, as we build a case for increased appropriations."[27]

In November 2007 the FDA issued a *Food Protection Plan*, which is an "integrated strategy for protecting the nation's food supply." The Plan offers three elements of protection. The first element is designed to prevent foodborne contamination: "promote increased corporate responsibility to prevent foodborne illness, identify food vulnerabilities and assess risks, and expand the understanding and use of effective mitigation measures." The second component involves intervention at "critical points in the food supply chain": "focused inspections and sampling based on risk, enhance risk-based surveillance, and improve the detection of food system 'signals' that indicate contamination." The final part focuses on the "rapid response to minimize harm": "improve immediate response and improve risk communications to the public, industry, and other stakeholders."[28]

The *Food Protection Plan* also calls for joining with Congress to make legislative changes in the FDA's authority. Among the requested changes are the following:

Prevent Foodborne Contamination.

Authorize FDA to issue additional preventive controls for high-risk foods.

Require food facilities to renew their FDA registration every two years, and allow FDA to modify registration categories.

Intervene at Critical Points in the Food Supply Chain.

Authorize FDA to accredit highly qualified third parties for voluntary food inspections.

Authorize FDA to require electronic import certificates for shipments of designated high-risk products.

Provide parity between domestic and imported foods if FDA inspection access is delayed, limited, or denied.

Respond Rapidly to Minimize Harm.

Empower FDA to issue a mandatory recall of food products when voluntary recalls are not effective.

Give FDA enhanced access to food records during emergencies.[29]

During January 29, 2008, testimony before the Subcommittee on Oversight and Investigations, Committee on Energy and Commerce, House of Representatives, Lisa Shames, the Director of Resources and Environment at the U.S. Government Accountability Office, agreed that the FDA needs more funding. Still, she said that the FDA needs to make better use of the resources that it has. In addition, Shames observed that the FDA's own Science Board, an advisory board to the agency, "concluded that the FDA is not positioned to meet current or emerging regulatory needs, and stated that [the] FDA does not have the capacity, such as staffing and technology, to ensure the safety of the nation's food supply."[30]

On the very same day, Andrew C. von Eschenbach, the FDA Commissioner of Food and Drugs, addressed the same Committee. Noting that the FDA has already "taken critical steps to begin to develop, articulate, and execute a well-designed plan for moving forward," von Eschenbach added that the "FDA is keenly aware that we must develop comprehensive solutions to face an ever-changing scientific and technological landscape. We look forward to working with Congress and other stakeholders to strengthen the scientific base at [the] FDA...."[31]

While the FDA attempts to provide better food safety protection for the American people, it may be useful to listen to suggestions from professionals who are well acquainted with the problems. During a September 2007 house hearing, Benjamin England and Carl Nielson, two former high-raking FDA regulators who now advise companies that export to the United States, said that the FDA has consistently failed to make necessary and long overdue changes. The greatest need, both men said, is "for a modernized information system that could integrate data from many sources to underpin risk analysis."[32] For example, England said that the system used to screen imports, which is called OASIS, is not integrated with other FDA systems. To determine the accuracy of information, much time is wasted entering and exiting databases. England said that the FDA must have systems that are "capable of receiving, integration and delivering data in a useful fashion to inspectors at the border."[33] In addition, England advised the FDA to move beyond a system focused on border inspections. The FDA must think in broader terms—"a food safety system based on regulatory equivalency in foreign countries and risk-based regulatory oversight in the U.S."[34]

At the same hearing, David Acheson, the FDA's Commissioner for Food Protection, called for a changing approach to food safety. At present, he said, the FDA examines food at the border. The borders must be extended. "To do that," he said, "we've got to get an understanding of what is going on at the manufacturing level in those countries."[35]

Meanwhile, in September 2007, Cal Dooley, the president and CEO of the Grocery Manufacturers Association, proposed the "Commitment to Consumers: The Four Pillars of Food Safety," a partnership between the government and private industry:

> Under pillar 1, all U.S. importers of record would be required to adopt a foreign supplier quality assurance program and verify that imported ingredients and products meet U.S. Food and Drug Administration (FDA) food safety and quality requirements. The program would be based on FDA guidance and industry best practices, and would be monitored and enforced by the FDA.[36]

The second pillar of the proposal would allow FDA to focus even greater resources on products and countries deemed of higher risk ... via a program that would allow food companies/importers to qualify their products as lower risk by sharing test results, data and supply chain information with the FDA in a confidential manner.[37] The third leg of the proposal focuses on building capacity within foreign governments so that as products move around the world there is a greater assurance of safety and quality.

Finally, recognizing that FDA must be armed with the appropriate resources to administer this program and adequately fulfill its food safety mission, the fourth pillar calls on the Administration and Congress to expand the capacity of FDA, providing the Agency with the resources it needs to get the job done.[38]

Dooley said that inspections alone are unable to provide the level of food safety that is needed. "Our industry can apply its vast knowledge and practical experience along the entire supply chain to prevent problems before they arise. And, under our proposal, a fortified FDA will be right there with us, side by side, to make sure we do it right."[39]

An article in the January 14, 2008, issue of *Nation's Restaurant News* agreed that the private sector could provide much needed overseas assistance. "Such inspections could serve as a proxy for FDA inspection. More importantly, private inspections can assist the FDA in focusing its inspection on imports with a higher risk."[40]

However this story plays out in the future remains to be seen. But it is quite evident that the time has come to raise the bar of prevention. Areas of concern must be identified before they result in outbreaks of illness. No one can afford to become complacent. Or else, the next outbreak is right around the corner—just waiting to happen.

CONCLUSION

Over the years, the amount of food that the United States imports has grown dramatically. This is because consumers, in general, want to be able to purchase items whenever they wish—whether or not they are in season. So if a consumer who lives in Maine wishes to purchase raspberries in January, they will be available. If one supermarket doesn't carry it, the next one certainly will.

Unfortunately, as the amount of imported food has risen, the amount of FDA inspectors needed to ensure the safety of this food has been reduced, and the resulting disease outbreaks have occurred.

Clearly, there is a need for a new food safety paradigm. Hopefully, the government and public industry will be able to work together to find better and more innovative solutions.

TOPICS FOR DISCUSSION

1. Have you ever been personally affected by a food recall? If so, describe what happened.

2. Have you ever stopped to think about the imported food you eat? What or why not? After reading this chapter do you think you should? Why or why not?

3. After reading this chapter, do you think you will be more careful about your food choices? Why or why not?

4. Do you think the FDA will be able to make the needed changes? Why or why not?

5. Do you think private industry should play an integral role in ensuring food safety?
Why or why not?

NOTES

1. "Imports from China Exploit Chaos in the U.S. Food Safety System," Comments of Caroline Smith DeWaal, Director of Food Safety, Center for Science in the Public Interest before the U.S. Senate Commerce Committee (July 18, 2007) 4, on website of Center for Science in the Public Interest, http://www.cspinet.org.

2. Linda Calvin, Belem Avendaño, and Rita Schwentesius, "The Economics of Food Safety: The Case of Green Onions and Hepatitis A Outbreaks," Economic Research Service, U.S. Department of Agriculture website, http://www.ers.usda.gov.

3. E. J. Mundell, "U.S. Food Safety: The Import Alarm Keeps Sounding," *U. S. News & World Report* (posted January 15, 2008) on HealthDay website, http://healthday.com.

4. "Imports from China Exploit Chaos in the U.S. Food Safety System," 5.

5. U. S. Food and Drug Administration website, http://www.fda.gov.

6. Margaret A. Handley, Celeste Hall, Eric Sanford, Evie Diaz, Enrique Gonzalez-Mendez, Kaitie Drace, Robert Wilson, Mario Villalobos, and Mary Croughan, "Globalization, Binational Communities, and Imported Food Risks: Results of an Outbreak Investigation of Lead Poisoning in Monterey County, California," *The American Journal of Public Health* (May 2007) 975): 900–6.

7. E. J. Mundell, "U.S. Food Safety: The Import Alarm Keeps Sounding."

8. Andrew Bridges, "Imported Food Rarely Inspected," *Washington Post* (April 16, 2007) NA.

9. Andrew Bridges, "Imported Food Rarely Inspected," NA.

10. Andrew Bridges, "Imported Food Rarely Inspected," NA.

11. Andrew Bridges, "Imported Food Rarely Inspected," NA.

12. E. J. Mundell, "U.S. Food Safety: The Import Alarm Keeps Sounding."

13. Matthew Enis, "Lack of Oversight," *Supermarket News* (October 15, 2007) 55(42): NA.

14. "Imports from China Exploit Chaos in the U.S. Food Safety System," 7.

15. Andrew Bridges, "Imported Food Rarely Inspected," NA.

16. Andrew Bridges and Seth Borenstein, "Food Safety; Yet Another Reason to Watch What You Eat; Oversight Agency Has Halved the Number of Inspections Over the Last Three Years," *The Houston Chronicle* (Houston, TX) (February 27, 2007) 1.

17. "U.S. Food Inspectors Overwhelmed by Imports," (April 23, 2007), http://www.msnbc.com/id/18271015.

18. "U.S. Food Inspectors Overwhelmed by Imports," (April 23, 2007).

19. Matthew Enis, Matthew, "Lack of Oversight," NA.

20. Marian Burros, "Who's Watching What We Eat?" *The New York Times* (May 16, 2007) F1.

21. Marian Burros, "Who's Watching What We Eat?" F1.

22. David M. Walker (Comptroller General of the United States), "Federal Oversight of Food Safety: High-Risk Designation Can Bring Needed Attention to Fragmented System." United States Government Accountability Office, Testimony Before the Subcommittee on Agriculture, Rural Development, FDA, and Related Agencies, Committee on Appropriates, House of Representatives (February 8, 2007) 12.

23. David M. Walker, "Federal Oversight of Food Safety: High Risk Designation Can Bring Needed Attention to Fragmented System," 12.

24. Coalition for a Stronger FDA website, http://www.fdacoalition.org.

25. Coalition for a Stronger FDA website.

26. Coalition for a Stronger FDA website.

27. Coalition for a Stronger FDA website.

28. U.S. Food and Drug Administration website.

29. U.S. Food and Drug Administration website.

30. Lisa Shames (Director, Natural Resources and Environment, U.S. Government Accountability Office), "Federal Oversight of Food Safety: FDA's Food Protection Plan Proposes Positive First Steps, but Capacity to Carry Them Out is Critical," Testimony Before the Subcommittee on Oversight and Investigations, Committee on Energy and Commerce, House of Representatives (January 29, 2008).

31. Andrew C. von Eschenbach (Commissioner of Food and Drugs, U.S. Food and Drug Administration), Statement Before Subcommittee on Oversight and Investigations, Committee on Energy and Commerce, U.S. House of Representatives (January 29, 2008) U.S. Food and Drug Administration website, http://www.fda.gov.

32. Sally Schuff, "FDA Flunks Exam at Imported Food Safety Hearing," *Foodstuffs* (October 1, 2007) 1–2.

33. Sally Schuff, "FDA Flunks Exam at Imported Food Safety Hearing," 1–2.

34. Sally Schuff, "FDA Flunks Exam at Imported Food Safety Hearing," 1–2.

35. Sally Schuff, "FDA Flunks Exam at Imported Food Safety Hearing," 1–2.

36. Grocery Manufacturers Association website, http://www.gmabrands.com.

37. "GMA Unveils Plan to Make Imported Food More Safe," *Progressive Grocer* (September 19, 2007) NA.

38. Grocery Manufacturers Association website.

39. "GMA Unveils Plan for Imported Food Safety," *Food Logistics* (October 15, 2007) 99: 10.

40. Aaron Krauss, "Private Inspections of Produce Can Help Alleviate the United States' Overburdened Border Control," *Nation's Restaurant News* (January 14, 2008) 42(2): 28.

REFERENCES AND RESOURCES

Magazines, Journals, and Newspapers

Bridges, Andrew. "Imported Food Rarely Inspected." *Washington Post* (April 16, 2007) NA.

Bridges, Andrew and Seth Borenstein. "Food Safety; Yet Another Reason to Watch What You Eat; Oversight Agency Has Halved Number of Inspections Over the Last Three Years." *The Houston Chronicle* (Houston, TX) (February 27, 2007) 1.

Burros, Marian. "Who's Watching What We Eat?" *The New York Times* (May 16, 2007) F1.

Enis, Matthew. "Lack of Oversight." *Supermarket News* (October 15, 2007) 55(42): NA.

"GMA Unveils Plan for Imported Food Safety." *Food Logistics* (October 15, 2007) 99: 10.

"GMA Unveils Plan to Make Imported Food More Safe." *Progressive Grocer* (September 19, 2007) NA.

Handley, Margaret A., Celeste Hall, Eric Sanford, Evie Diaz, Enrique Gonzalez-Mendez, Kaitie Drace, Robert Wilson, Mario Villalobos, and Mary Croughan. "Globalization, Binational Communities, and Imported Food Risks: Results of an Outbreak Investigation of Lead Poisoning in Monterey County, California." *The American Journal of Public Health* (May 2007) 95(5): 900–906.

Krauss, Aaron. "Private Inspections of Produce Can Help Alleviate the United States' Overburdened Border Control." *Nation's Restaurant News* (January 14, 2008) 42(2): 28.

"Multistate Outbreaks of *Salmonella* Serotype Poona Infections Associated with Eating Cantaloupe from Mexico—United States and Canada, 2000–2002." *MMWR Weekly* (November 22, 2002) 51(46): 1044–1047.

Mundell, E. J. "U.S. Food Safety: The Import Alarm Keeps Sounding." *U. S. News & World Report* (posted January 15, 2008) on HealthDay website, http://healthday.com.

Schuff, Sally. "FDA Flunks Exam at Imported Food Safety Hearing." *Foodstuffs* (October 1, 2007) 1–2.

Shames, Lisa (Director, Natural Resources and Environment, U.S. Government Accountability Office). "Federal Oversight of Food Safety: FDA's Food Protective Plan Proposes Positive First Steps, But Capacity to Carry Them Out Is Critical." United States Government Accountability Office, Testimony Before the Subcommittee on Oversight and Investigations, Committee on Energy and Commerce, House of Representatives, January 29, 2008.

"U.S. Food Inspectors Overwhelmed By Imports." (April 23, 2007), www.msnbc.com/id/18271015.

United States Government Accountability Office, Testimony Before the Subcommittee on Agriculture, Rural Development, FDA, and Related Agencies, Committee on Appropriations, House of Representatives, February 8, 2007.

Walker, David M (Comptroller General of the United States). "Federal Oversight of Food Safety: High-Risk Designation Can Bring Needed Attention to Fragmented System."

Websites

Alliance for a Stronger FDA
http://www.StrengthenFDA.org

Center for Science in the Public Interest
http://www.cspinet.org

Coalition for a Stronger FDA
http://www.fdacoalition.org

Economic Research Service
U.S. Department of Agriculture
http://www.ers.usda.gov

Grocery Manufacturers Association
http://www.gmabrands.com

U.S. Food and Drug Administration
http://www.fda.gov

U. S. Government Accountability Office
http://www.gao.gov

Chapter 11

Life-Enhancing/Life-Threatening Foods

Not all food is healthful. Some is downright dangerous, and it is not always evident which is which. A clear and undeniable correlation exists between food and illness. Eating certain foods on a regular basis will tend to make you healthier. It is not surprising that other foods have the opposite effect. Eating too many of these may well have long-term negative consequences. Foods may be deceptive. Something may appear to be healthful when, in fact, it is not. Another food may seem to be a poor choice, when it's actually a better alternative.

Even the healthiest foods may carry a foodborne disease if they are handled improperly or inadequately prepared. Such foods have the potential to cause serious illness or death. There are also people who have food allergies and intolerances. For them, the ingestion of seemingly harmless items may have profoundly negative effects. Then there are "miracle" foods that are believed to help heal a variety of medical problems. The relationship between food and well-being is far more complicated than it may initially appear to be.

DEPARTMENT OF AGRICULTURE DIETARY RECOMMENDATIONS

"Dietary Guidelines for Americans 2005," which is published by the U.S. Department of Agriculture, presents a number of principles that may be useful in the food selection process. For the average person, who should have a daily intake of about 2,000 calories, the diet should include about two cups of fruit and two and one-half cups of vegetables. It is best to include many different types of fruits and vegetables. In addition, "consume 3 or more ounce-equivalents of whole-grain products per day, with the rest of the recommended grains coming from enriched or whole-grain products. In general, at least half the

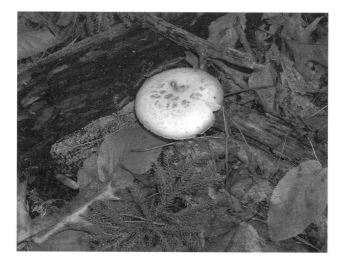

Wild mushrooms may be life-threatening. (Courtesy of Mark A. Goldstein)

grains should come from whole grains."[1] As for dairy, the guidelines advise three cups per day of fat-free or low-fat milk or equivalent milk products.

How about fats? The guidelines suggest less than 10 percent of all calories should come from saturated fats and fewer than 300 milligrams per day from cholesterol-rich foods. Trans fat should be kept as low as possible. Total fat intake should be between 20 and 35 percent of total calories. Most fat intake should be from sources of polyunsaturated and monounsaturated fats. These include fish, nuts, and vegetable oils. "When selecting and preparing meat, poultry, dry beans, and milk or milk products, makes choices that are lean, low-fat, or fat-free."[2]

Thus, the guidelines acknowledge that there are differences in types of fat. Saturated fats are likely to raise blood cholesterol. They are found in high-fat dairy products, fatty fresh and processed meats, the skin and fat of poultry, lard, palm oil, and coconut oil. Foods high in cholesterol, such as liver and other organ meats, egg yolks, and dairy fats, also tend to raise blood cholesterol, as do trans fats (also known as trans fatty acids). Trans fats are found in shortening and many hard types of margarines, which are common ingredients in some commercially fried foods and some bakery goods.

Unsaturated fats (oils), which do not raise blood cholesterol, are found in vegetable oils, most nuts, olives, avocadoes, and fatty fish like salmon. Olive, canola, sunflower, and peanut oils are high in monounsaturated fats. Soybean and corn oils and many kinds of nuts are sources of polyunsaturated fats. (See Chapter 4.)

The following U.S. Department of Agriculture table compares the saturated fat content of some foods:

Food	Amount	Saturated Fat Content (grams)
Cheese		
Regular cheddar cheese	1 oz	6.0
Low-fat cheddar cheese	1 oz	1.2
Ground Beef		
Regular ground beef (25% fat)	3 oz cooked	6.1
Extra lean ground beef (5% fat)	3 oz cooked	2.6
Milk		
Whole milk (3.5% fat)	1 cup	4.6
Low-fat (1% fat)	1 cup	1.5
Breads		
Croissant	1 medium	6.6
Bagel, oat bran	1 medium	0.2
Frozen Desserts		
Regular ice cream	1/2 cup	4.9
Frozen yogurt, low-fat	1/2 cup	2.0
Table Spreads		
Butter	1 tsp	2.4
Soft margarine with zero trans fat	1 tsp	0.7
Chicken		
Fried chicken (leg, with skin)	3 oz cooked	3.3
Roasted chicken (breast, no skin)	3 oz cooked	0.9
Fish		
Fried fish	3 oz	2.8
Baked fish	3 oz	1.5[3]

It is important to remember that fat content may be difficult to detect. Although it is obvious that foods such as butter, cream, and margarine contain fat, fat may also be found in foods such as cookies, peanut butter, and crackers. Most restaurant foods are known to be higher in fat.

Sugar

Like fat, dietary sugars should be limited. In the United States, the major sources of added sugar are soft drinks, cakes, cookies, pies, drinks such as punch and lemonade, dairy desserts, and candy. Added sugar comes in a variety of forms and under names such as brown sugar, corn sweetener, corn syrup, dextrose, and fructose. The excess consumption of foods containing high amount of sugars may easily lead to weight gain, and it may reduce the consumption of more nutritious foods. Moreover, when there are higher amounts of sugar in the bloodstream, the pancreas releases more insulin. Insulin then increases the release of the lipoprotein lipase, an enzyme that facilities the transfer of fat from the bloodstream into fat cells. When fat is in the cells, it is more difficult to remove. Furthermore, insulin plays a direct role in the production of cholesterol. Higher levels of circulating insulin result in the production of more cholesterol by the liver. There is also some indication that insulin levels help determine where an individual stores excess body fat. People with higher levels of insulin tend to have more abdominal weight gain, which is the type of weight gain associated with cardiac disease.

Salt

There should be similar constraints on the intake of salt. Most people are advised to consume no more than 2,400 milligrams of sodium, or about a teaspoon, per day, of salt. People over the age of fifty should consume no more than 1,500 milligrams. Often, the problem is not the added salt from the salt shaker but the salt contained in processed foods. The following are some of the major sources of dietary sodium: soy sauce, frozen dinners, canned soups, processed meats, pickles, relishes, and olives. In *Eating Between the Lines*, which was published in 2007, Kimberly Lord Stewart describes how a person's daily intake of salt may quickly climb. "Breakfast: instant oatmeal with brown sugar cinnamon (325 mg), 1/2 cup juice-packed canned peaches (5 mg); lunch: turkey sandwich on whole-wheat bread (1,800 mg), 1/2 cup tomato soup (713 mg); dinner: green salad with fat-free bottle Italian salad dressing (280 mg), broiled chicken breast with a pinch of salt (150 mg), 1/2 canned corn with 1/2 tab. butter (220 mg); dessert: mint chip no-sugar, light ice cream (50 mg)."[4] That's a total of 3,543 milligrams for the day.

According to the author, with a few modifications the salt content may be lowered. These include "regular oatmeal (2 mg), lower-sodium roast turkey (430 mg), low-salt tomato soup (90 mg), and a green salad with homemade vinegar EVOO [extra virgin olive oil] dressing (0 mg)."[5] The sodium content has been reduced to 947 milligrams.

One way to remove some of the salt is to rinse canned foods. So, before making tuna salad, place the tuna in a strainer and rinse for a few seconds. Also remember that salt may appear in foods under different names including sodium nitrate, sodium citrate, monosodium glutamate, sodium phosphate, and sodium saccharin.[6]

AMERICAN HEART ASSOCIATION GUIDELINES

The American Heart Association (AHA) offers a number of suggestions for adhering to a healthful diet. According to the AHA, people should begin by determining how many calories they should consume each day:

Gender	Age (years)	Activity Level and Estimated Calories Burned		
		Sedentary	Moderately Active	Active
Female	19–30	2,000	2,000–2,200	2,400
	31–50	1,800	2,000	2,200
	51+	1,600	1,800	2,000–2,200
Male	19–30	2,400	2,600–2,800	3,000
	31–50	2,200	2,400–2,600	2,800–3,000
	51+	2,000	2,200–2,400	2,400–2,800

Sedentary: Sedentary means you have a lifestyle that includes only the light physical activity associated with typical day-to-day life.

Moderately Active: Moderately active means you have a lifestyle that includes physical activity equivalent to walking about 1.5 to 3 miles per day at 3 to 4 miles per hour, in addition to the physical activity associated with typical day-to-day life.

Active: Active means you have a lifestyle that includes physical activity equivalent to walking more than 3 miles per day at 3 to 4 miles per hour, in addition to the light physical activity associated with typical day-to-day life.[7]

The AHA notes that a nutrient-rich diet includes fruits, vegetables, unrefined whole-grain foods, and fish, at least twice per week. Additional guidelines are as follows:

- Choose lean meats and poultry without skin and prepare them without added saturated and trans fat.
- Select fat-free 1 percent fat, and low-fat dairy products.
- Cut back on foods containing partially hydrogenated vegetable oils to reduce trans fat in your diet.
- Cut back on foods high in dietary cholesterol. Aim to eat less than 300 milligrams of cholesterol each day.
- Cut back on beverages and foods with added sugars.

- Choose and prepare foods with little or no salt. Aim to eat less than 2,300 milligrams of sodium per day.
- If you drink alcohol, drink in moderation. That means one drink per day if you're a woman and two drinks per day if you're a man.[8]

THE MEDITERRANEAN DIET

Mediterranean populations are known to have lower rates of heart disease and some cancers than people in the United States. The diet, which includes lots of fruits and vegetables, fish, whole grains, olive oil, and a daily glass of wine, has low intakes of cholesterol as well as saturated and polyunsaturated fats. A 2008 article in *U. S. News & World Report* noted that this diet needs to be coupled with an active lifestyle. "Men in post-war Crete didn't laze around dunking bread in olive oil all day; they chased goats up hills. Even now, people in the Mediterranean and other parts of the world are more active, whether through vocation or because there's so much more walking as part of daily life."[9]

A study published in 2006 in the *Annals of Internal Medicine* examined the short-term effects of two Mediterranean diets versus those of a low-fat diet. In total, there were 772 asymptomatic people between the ages of fifty-five and eighty who were considered at high risk for cardiovascular disease. At the end of three months, the researchers found, "compared with a low-fat diet, [the] Mediterranean diets supplemented with olive oil or nuts have beneficial effects on cardiovascular risk factors." Moreover, the extra "healthy fat" contained in the Mediterranean diet did not result in weight gain.[10]

In a National Institutes of Health/AARP (formerly known as American Association of Retired Persons) study of 214,284 men and 166,012 women, which was published in 2007 in the *Annals of Internal Medicine*, researchers examined the association between the Mediterranean diet and death. The results found that those who followed the Mediterranean diet had a reduced "risk of death from all causes, including deaths due to CVD [cardiovascular disease] and cancer, in a US population."[11]

In the book, *The Mediterranean Diet*, which was published in 2006, authors Marissa Cloutier and Eve Adamson explain that because the diet features low calorie, high-fiber foods, it may even be a means to drop some pounds. "Design your meals to feature fresh produce and whole grains. Use high-fat animal products only occasionally, deriving daily protein from beans, low-fat dairy products (or preferably low-fat soy products, such as low-fat soy milk), moderate amounts of nuts, and small amounts of low-fat meat for flavoring. Stick to single portions, and add to that a more active lifestyle. You should be able to lose weight, if you are overweight, with relative ease."[12]

FOOD CONTAMINATION

Sometimes perfectly healthful food, such as produce, becomes contaminated. A 2005 article in *Environmental Nutrition* says that, "In recent years, numerous microbes have made their way onto fresh fruits and vegetables. In the late 1990s, raspberries from Guatemala contaminated with the Cyclospora parasite gave nearly 1,400 people diarrhea. A few years later, Salmonella-tainted cantaloupes wreaked havoc, while just last summer, Salmonella on Roma tomatoes was to blame for making more than 600 people sick in the U.S. and Canada. And in perhaps one of the worst cases of produce contamination, Mexican-grown scallions were guilty of transmitting the hepatitis A virus to diners a few years back."[13] There are many ways for this to happen. Wild animals and birds may contaminate produce on a farm with their feces. Water from wells or streams and rainwater runoff may foul crops. Manure from cattle or poultry may contain pathogens.

Of course, humans are also a source of contamination. Humans who handle produce during harvesting may spread human pathogens such as hepatitis A or transfer contaminated dirt on to the produce. Processing facilities may be vulnerable to contamination from dust or animals. Dirt floors and unclean water are further risks.

An article published in 2006 in *Healthy Eating (Harvard Special Health Report)* maintains that contamination is very much part of modern farming and food-processing methods. "Efforts to maximize yield have led to greater use of pesticides on crops and hormones in animals. The crowded animal pens of factory farms and the large-scale assembly-line nature of slaughterhouses and food processing plants have increased the spread of dangerous bacteria in food."[14]

This article contends that the biggest threat is from bacterial contamination, a concern for meat, fish, dairy products, and some fresh produce. "Microbes that not long ago were either unheard of or considered a minor threat now cause 76 million cases of food poisoning and 5,000 deaths in the United States each year."[15] The author believes that this is primarily caused by the increasing use of antibiotics in animal feed that has triggered disease-resistant pathogens, "superbugs," that are resistant to antibiotics. "These resistant germs breed inside the animals and are then passed to humans in meat, eggs, and other foods." Because modern farms tend to be large, when contamination occurs, it has the potential to affect large amounts of food that has been shipped to supermarkets, restaurants, and school cafeterias.[16]

A study published in 2001 in the *New England Journal of Medicine* showed the prevalence of Salmonella, which is mostly found in meat and eggs but may spread to other foods, including fruit and ice cream. Of 200 samples of chicken, beef, turkey, and pork, 20 percent were found to contain Salmonella. Eighty-four percent of the Salmonella were resistant to at least one antibiotic; 53 percent were resistant to at least three antibiotics. Because of this resistance, people who become ill from Salmonella will be harder to treat. The researchers concluded that guidelines need to be adopted for "the prudent use of antibiotics in food animals and for a reduction in the number of pathogens present on farms and in slaughterhouses. National surveillance for antimicrobial-resistant Salmonella should be extended to include retail meats."[17]

An editorial in the same issue of *New England Journal of Medicine* explained that antimicrobials, such as penicillin and tetracycline, have been used in feed animals for about half a century. As a result, one study determined that at least 17 percent of chickens sold in supermarkets in four states contained campylobacter strains that were resistant to antibiotics. Campylobacter is a bacterium that is frequently seen in poultry. Although it is often stated that such antimicrobials are needed for efficiency and economic savings, the author disagrees. When European countries stopped using these drugs, they found that the "economic losses could be minimized and even neutralized by improvements in animal husbandry, the quality of feed, and hygiene."[18]

SUGGESTED PRECAUTIONS

Though it is probably impossible to avoid all food-related illnesses, by following a few practices at home, it is possible to reduce the risk. The government website www.FoodSafety.gov shares a few suggestions:

When Shopping:
Separate raw meat, poultry, and seafood from other foods in your grocery-shopping cart. Place these foods in plastic bags to prevent their juices from dripping onto other foods. It is also best to separate these foods from other foods at check out and in your grocery bags.

When Refrigerating Food:
Place raw meat, poultry, and seafood in containers or sealed plastic bags to prevent their juices from dripping onto other foods. Raw juices often contain harmful bacteria. Store eggs in their original carton, and refrigerate as soon as possible.

When Preparing Food:
Wash hands and surfaces often. Harmful bacteria can spread throughout the kitchen and get onto cutting boards, utensils, and counter tops.

Cutting Boards:
Always use a clean cutting board. If possible, use one cutting board for fresh produce and a separate one for raw meat, poultry, and seafood. Once cutting boards become excessively worn or develop hard-to-clean groves, you should replace them.

Marinating Food:

Always marinate food in the refrigerator, not on the counter. Sauce that is used to marinate raw meat, poultry, or seafood should not be used on cooked foods, unless it is boiled just before using.

When Serving Food:

Always use a clean plate. Never placed cooked food back on the same plate or cutting board that previously held raw food.

When Storing Leftovers:

Refrigerate or freeze leftovers within 2 hours or sooner in clean, shallow, covered containers to prevent harmful bacteria from multiplying.[19]

Following the 40-140 rule is a good way to keep food safe. Keeping hot foods above 140 degrees and cold foods below 40 degrees prevents most bacteria from multiplying. Hot leftovers should be refrigerated quickly, preferably in a container with a large surface area to promote fast cooling. Foods left out in the open between 40 and 140 degrees are fertile breeding grounds for bacteria and viruses. Keep foods between these temperatures for no longer than two hours, and be especially careful with such protein foods as ham, chicken, and egg salad.

Despite the problems, there is still a measure of control within the home setting. When people eat away from home, as they so often do, that control is gone. According to the National Restaurant Association, in 2008, $558 billion was spent in restaurant sales. In the United States there are about 945,000 restaurants that employ 13.1 million people. On a typical day in 2008, restaurant industry sales were $1.5 billion.

In *It Was Probably Something You Ate,* which was published in 1999, Nicols Fox wrote, "When you eat away from home, the safety of your food is in someone else's hands.... And those hands, in all probability, belong to someone making minimum wage, who doesn't have sick leave either. You cannot be sure they are clean hands, or that the person they are connected to has had any training in food safety, or even that the restaurant owner has as clear understanding of how foodborne microbes get into food. In short, eating out, from a food-safety perspective, involves risk."[20]

Nevertheless, there are ways to reduce the risk when eating in a restaurant. According to Barbara Sheen, the author of *Food Poisoning*, which was published in 2005, whenever possible, people should avoid eating raw fish, such as the raw fish in sushi and raw oysters. Salad bars are also problematic. "Foods on a salad bar or buffet may not be kept cold or warm enough, allowing bacteria to grow. Customers may also spread infection by touching items on the salad bar or buffet with their bare hands or sneezing or coughing on the food items. In addition, customers often cause cross-contamination by switching utensils that are provided for individual items on a buffet."[21]

FOOD ALLERGIES AND INTOLERANCES

There are still other ways in which food may make us ill. Some people have allergies and/or intolerances to foods. An allergic response is an adverse reaction of the body's immune system to even a tiny amount of a particular food (usually some form of protein) or an environmental agent such as an animal enzyme or plant pollen. Allergic reactions are out of proportion to the amount of alien material taken into the body and may even be fatal. On the other hand, an intolerance response takes place when the body is unable to "detoxify" certain elements of something that is ingested. There is no involvement of the immune system. In *Dealing with Food Allergies in Babies and Children*, which was published in 2007, Janice Vickerstaff Joneja wrote, "Most intolerance reactions that we understand (and there are many that we do not!) involve a defect in the processing of the food, either during digestion, or later, after the food parts, or components, have been absorbed into the body. The symptoms of food intolerance are often caused by an excess of a component that has not been digested completely (for example, lactose intolerance) or a component that, for some reason, cannot be processed efficiently after it has entered the body."[22]

Allergic reactions may be immediate and intense or develop over a relatively brief period of time. Intolerances are generally slower in coming. About 90 percent of food allergies are caused by eight types of foods: dairy, eggs, fish, shellfish, tree nuts, wheat, peanuts, and soybeans. In *Hidden Food Allergies*, which was published in 2006, James Braly and Patrick Holford note that cow's milk is the most frequent food allergen. "Most cheeses, cream, yogurt, and butter contain milk protein, and it's hidden in all sorts of food. If you check labels, you'll find it's sometimes called simple milk protein, sometimes whey (which is milk protein with the casein removed), and sometimes casein or caseinate, which is the predominant type of protein—and the most allergenic—in dairy products."[23]

In *Food Allergies and Food Intolerance*, which was published in 2000, Jonathan Brostoff and Linda Gamlin describe the experience of Jane, a person with an allergy to peanuts. When Jane was a child, her mouth and tongue swelled enormously on one or two occasions, and she had to be rushed to the hospital. Her mother concluded that peanuts were the cause, and prick tests confirmed the diagnosis. Jane carefully avoided peanuts, but one day, when she was about eight, she handed a bowl of nuts to the guests at a party her parents were giving. Later, she rubbed her eyelids, and they began to swell and itch. Years later, Jane had a career that involved a good deal of traveling and eating out. On one occasion, she ordered some cheesecake. The waiter assured her that the brown powder on the dessert was pure chocolate. Unfortunately, the supply of chocolate had run out, and the chef has used finely grated nuts, including peanuts. As soon as Jane ate her first bite of cheesecake, her mouth began to itch. Her tongue swelled and blocked her windpipe. She soon collapsed on the floor. A doctor happened to be at the next table, and he managed to unblock her windpipe. Someone else telephoned the hospital, and another doctor brought the lifesaving medicines Jane needed.[24]

Brostoff and Gamlin note some of the common symptoms of food intolerance: headache, migraine, fatigue, depression/anxiety, hyperactivity (in children), recurrent mouth ulcers, aching muscles, vomiting, nausea, stomach ulcers, duodenal ulcers, diarrhea, constipation, flatulence, bloating, joint pain, and edema (water retention).[25] Frequently, the offending food may be detected with an elimination diet or a diet in which specific foods are removed from the diet for several days. If the person's health improves, then he or she may well have one or more food intolerances.

At least a portion of the people who suffer from food intolerance probably have celiac disease, an autoimmune disorder in which the body cannot tolerate gluten, a protein found in wheat, oats (through cross-contamination), barley, and rye. Not that long ago, celiac disease was thought to be a rare medical problem. The National Institutes of Health (NIH) Celiac Disease Awareness Campaign now estimates that about one percent of all Americans have this disorder, "though many have never been diagnosed and are not receiving treatment."[26] In their previously noted book, James Braly and Patrick Holford wrote that as many as one in 100 people may have celiac disease, "often showing no digestive symptoms as all."[27] "The incidence is higher in those with gastrointestinal symptoms—1 in 40 children and 1 in 30 adults."[28]

When people with celiac disease eat gluten, the gluten damages the fingerlike protrusions in the lining of the small intestine (villi). Normally, nutrients from food are absorbed through these villi. Without the villi, absorption is disrupted, and people may easily become malnourished. In *Food Allergies*, which was published in 2000, William E. Walsh notes that celiac disease is different from food allergies. Although they may have a devastating effect on the body, food allergies do not harm body tissues. "In gluten-sensitive people, it [gluten] strips away the inner layer of the intestine like sandpaper. The 'sandpapered' intestine handles food poorly; it struggles to absorb the proteins, carbohydrates, and vitamins from food, and this poor absorption can lead to malnutrition. It poorly absorbs water and other dietary components necessary for health. Much of what a sufferer eats and drinks passes through the intestine and ends up uselessly in the stool."[29]

Because celiac disease is genetically linked, it tends to run in families. According to the National Foundation for Celiac Awareness, "Among people who have a first-degree relative diagnosed with celiac, as many as 1 in 22 may have the disease."[30] It may appear in childhood or anytime in adulthood. Even elderly people are diagnosed. It is not at all uncommon for the disease to be triggered by pregnancy, childbirth, surgery, a viral infection, or serious emotional upset. The Foundation says that the following are some of the most common symptoms:

- Bloating or gas
- Itchy skin rash
- Diarrhea
- Constipation
- Fatigue
- Tingling/numbness
- Pale mouth sores
- Joint pain
- Delayed growth
- Poor weight gain
- Thin bones
- Infertility
- Headaches
- Depression
- Irritability
- Discolored teeth[31]

The Foundation notes that anemia, delayed growth, and weight loss are all signs of malnutrition. "Malnutrition is a serious problem for anyone, but particularly for children because they need adequate nutrition to develop properly. Failure to thrive during childhood development is a common indicator of celiac."[32]

Many celiacs do not have noticeable symptoms. This is called asymptomatic celiac disease. "The undamaged part of their small intestine is able to absorb enough nutrients to prevent symptoms. However, people without symptoms are still at risk for the complications of celiac disease."[33] And celiacs have an increased risk for developing another autoimmune disorder, such as diabetes or thyroid disease.

Testing for celiac disease usually begins by determining the levels of antibodies to gluten contained in the blood. If the tests are positive, physicians may decide to use a long, thin tube, known as an endoscope, to take tissue samples from the small intestine.

Celiac disease is treated by following a gluten-free diet. This is not as easy as it may initially appear to be. Gluten is not only found in obvious foods, such as bread and pasta, but it is hidden in a host of prepared foods, such as salad dressings and soups. It is also found in some medications and supplements. After being diagnosed with celiac disease, people need to read labels carefully, and, when in doubt, they should not hesitate to telephone a manufacturer. If the manufacturer is unable to help, the product should be avoided. Most certainly, there is an alternative. Cosmetic products, like lipsticks, may also contain gluten.

In *Kids with Celiac Disease*, which was published in 2001, Danna Korn, the mother of a child with celiac disease and founder of Raising Our Celiac Kids (ROCK), an international support group, listed some additional items of possible unease:

- Rice and soy beverages, because their production process utilizes barley enzymes
- Bad advice from health-food-store employees (e.g., that spelt is safe for celiacs)
- Cross-contamination between bins in food stores selling raw flours and grains (usually via the scoops)
- Wheat-bread crumbs in butter and jams, in the toaster, on the counter, and the like
- Stamps, envelopes, or other gummed labels
- Toothpaste and mouthwash
- Medicines, many of which contain gluten
- Cereals, most of which contain malt flavoring or some other non-gluten-free ingredient
- Some brands of rice paper
- Sauce mixes and sauces, such as soy sauce, fish sauce, catsup, mustard, and mayonnaise
- Ice cream
- Packet and canned soups
- Dried meals and gravy mixes
- Laxatives
- Grilled restaurant food, because the grill may be contaminated with gluten
- Fried restaurant food, because the grease may be contaminated
- Ground spices, in which wheat flour is commonly used to prevent clumping[34]

In *The Gluten Connection*, which was published in 2007, Shari Lieberman offers several suggestions for eating in restaurants. Some of these are as follows:

- Have a snack before you go.
- Tell your server you have a 'wheat allergy.'

- Bypass fried food.
- Stick to plain protein, potatoes or rice, and vegetables.
- Order naked salads.
- Use only oil and vinegar salad dressing.
- Substitute rice, beans, lentils, or potatoes for pasta.[35]

HEALING FOODS

There are foods that are naturally healing. Although it is impossible to note all of them, it may be useful to mention a few. In *Super Feast*, which was published in 2005, Michael van Straten discusses the potential benefits of a number of foods. One of these is broccoli, which is a cruciferous vegetable that has been proven to have protective powers against cancer, especially colorectal cancer. "Six out of seven major population studies showed that the more cruciferous vegetables you eat, the lower your chances of developing cancer of the colon. Other cancers appeared to slow down as well."[36]

Cranberries are another of van Straten's healing foods. Native to North America, they have been used for centuries as both food and medicine. Native Americans would wash injuries with cranberry juice and place cranberry poultices on wounds. In today's world, they are commonly used to prevent problems such as cystitis. "Cranberries contain substances that stick to the lining of the bladder, kidney and internal plumbing, and they stop bacteria from making their home in these sensitive tissues."[37]

Still another of van Straten's favorites is garlic, which has been used since ancient times as a medicinal plant. Garlic is believed to be useful for such disparate medical problems as constipation, diarrhea, bronchitis, sore throat, asthma, and athlete's foot. But it is probably best known for supporting heart and circulatory health. "The sulphur compound allicin, released when garlic is crushed, both encourages the elimination of cholesterol from the body, and reduces the quantity of unhealthy fats produced by the liver."[38]

A 2008 article in *Natural Life* highlights some of the healing powers of ginger. Many generations of people have used ginger for nausea, upset stomach, motion sickness, and the loss of appetite. But more recent research has found that it may well inhibit the growth of colorectal cancer cells. "In 2006, researchers from the University of Michigan Comprehensive Cancer Center found that ginger not only kills cancer cells, it also prevents them from building up resistance to cancer treatment."[39] And in a study published in 2007 in *BMC Complementary and Alternative*, researchers examined the role that ginger may play in the prevention and treatment of ovarian cancer. When they treated cultured ovarian cancer cells with ginger, they found significant growth inhibition. The researchers concluded that, "ginger inhibits growth and modulates secretion of angiogenic [the making of new blood vessels] factors in ovarian cancer cells."[40]

A 2008 article in *Vegetarian Times*, entitled "Healing Foods," describes the healing powers of medicinal mushrooms—maitake, shitake, reishi, and the common white button mushroom. These mushrooms contain significant amounts of dietary fibers that lower cholesterol and boost the immune system. "The mushrooms also offer high-quality protein, vitamins, and healthful unsaturated fatty acids. Medicinal mushrooms have been used for 2,000 years in Asia to treat an array of ailments and ward off disease. More scientific studies are needed, but initial findings suggest they support heart health, reduce cancer risk, and more."[41]

CONCLUSION

It is not always clear which foods are healthful and which are not. A food that may be beneficial for one person has the potential to harm or even kill another. What could be wrong with a slice of whole wheat toast? Nutritionists have been telling us to eat whole wheat products for years. Yet a person with celiac disease may become quite ill from even trace amounts of wheat. And what could be wrong with a single peanut? For someone with a peanut allergy, it could be deadly. Every day, people become sick from food that is not handled properly. It is important for people to educate themselves on the ways to ensure the safe handling of food. On the other hand, there are foods that appear to be natural healers. Although more medical research needs to be conducted on these, they should be included in diets as often as possible.

TOPICS FOR DISCUSSION

1. Do you believe that there is a strong correlation between diet and illness? Why or why not?
2. Should you be concerned if your diet is high in fat, sugar, or salt? Why or why not?
3. Do you take steps to keep your home-cooked food safer? What are some of the things that you do?
4. Do you take steps to avoid food poisoning when you eat in restaurants? If so, what do you do?
5. Do you believe in the power of healing foods? Why or why not?

NOTES

1. U.S. Department of Agriculture website, http://www.usda.gov.
2. U.S. Department of Agriculture website.

3. U.S. Department of Agriculture website.

4. Kimberly Lord Stewart, *Eating Between the Lines* (New York: St. Martin's Press, 2007) 222.

5. Kimberly Lord Stewart, *Eating Between the Lines*, 222.

6. Kimberly Lord Stewart, *Eating Between the Lines*, 223.

7. American Heart Association website, http://www.americanheart.org.

8. American Heart Association website.

9. Katherine Hobson, "'Diets' That Promote Health (and Always Have); Giving Up Their Hunt For Charmed Nutrients, Diet Experts Increasingly Embrace Whole Patterns of Eating," *U. S. News and World Report* (April 7, 2008) NA.

10. Ramon Estruch, Miguel Angel Martinez-González, Dolores Corella, et al., "Effects of a Mediterranean-Style Diet on Cardiovascular Risk Factors," *Annals of Internal Medicine* (July 4, 2006) 145: 1–11.

11. Panagiota N. Mitrou, Victor Kipnis, Anne C. M. Thiébaut, et al., "Mediterranean Dietary Pattern and Prediction of All-Cause Mortality in a US Population," *Archives of Internal Medicine* (December 10/24, 2007) 2461–8.

12. Marissa Cloutier and Eve Adamson, *Mediterranean Diet* (New York: HarperCollins, 2006) 32.

13. Elizabeth M. Ward, "Suspect Produce: How to be Safe from Contaminated Fruits, Vegetables," *Environmental Nutrition* (June 2005) 28: 1.

14. Frank M. Sacks, "How Safe is Your Food?" *Healthy Eating (Harvard Special Health Report)* (February 2006) 37.

15. Frank M. Sacks, "How Safe is Your Food?" 37.

16. Frank M. Sacks, "How Safe is Your Food?" 37.

17. David G. White, Shaohua Zhao, Robert Sudler, et al., "The Isolation of Antibiotic-Resistant Salmonella from Retail Ground Meats," *New England Journal of Medicine* (October 18, 2001) 345: 1147–54.

18. Sherwood L. Gorbach, "Antimicrobial Use in Animal Feed–Time to Stop," *New England Journal of Medicine* (October 18, 2001) 345: 1202–3.

19. http://www.FoodSafety.gov.

20. Nicols Fox, *It Was Probably Something You Ate* (New York: Penguin Books, 1999) 127.

21. Barbara Sheen, *Food Poisoning* (Farmington, Michigan: Lucent Books, 2005) 59.

22. Janice Vickerstaff Joneja, *Dealing with Food Allergies in Babies and Children* (Boulder, Colorado: Bull Publishing Company, 2007) 2.

23. James Braly and Patrick Holford, *Hidden Food Allergies* (Laguna Beach, California: Basic Health Publications, Inc., 2006) 58.

24. Jonathan Brostoff and Linda Gamlin, *Food Allergies and Food Intolerance* (Rochester, Vermont: Healing Arts Press, 2000) 1–2.

25. Jonathan Brodstoff and Linda Gamlin, *Food Allergies and Food Intolerance*, 15.

26. National Institute of Diabetes and Digestive and Kidney Diseases website, http://www2.niddk.nih.gov.

27. James Braly and Patrick Holford, *Hidden Food Allergies*, 62.

28. James Braly and Patrick Holford, *Hidden Food Allergies*, 62.

29. William E. Walsh, *Food Allergies* (New York: John Wiley and Sons, 2000).

30. National Foundation for Celiac Awareness website, www.celiaccentral.org.

31. National Foundation for Celiac Awareness website.

32. National Foundation for Celiac Awareness website.

33. National Foundation for Celiac Awareness website.

34. Danna Korn, *Kids with Celiac Disease* (Bethesda, Maryland: Woodbine House, 2001) 66.

35. Shari Lieberman with Linda Segall, *The Gluten Connection* (Emmaus, Pennsylvania, and New York: Rodale, 2007) 118–9.

36. Michael van Straten, *Super Feast* (London: Little Books Ltd., 2005) 43.

37. Michael van Straten, *Super Feast*, 54.

38. Michael van Straten, *Super Feast*, 60.

39. "Ginger and Cancer," *Natural Life* (March–April, 2008) 36.

40. Jennifer Rhode, Sarah Fogoros, Suzanna Zick, et al., "Ginger Inhibits Cell Growth and Modulates Angiogenic Factors in Ovarian Cancer Cells," *BMC Complementary and Alternative Medicine* (December 20, 2007) 7: 44.

41. Matthew Solan, "Healing Foods," *Vegetarian Times* (September 2008) 34(8): 30–2.

REFERENCES AND RESOURCES

Books

Braley, James and Patrick Holford. *Hidden Food Allergies.* Laguna Beach, California: Basic Health Publications, Inc., 2006.

Brostoff, Jonathan and Linda Gamlin. *Food Allergies and Food Intolerance.* Rochester, Vermont: Healing Arts Press, 2000.

Cloutier, Marissa and Eve Adamson. *The Mediterranean Diet.* New York: HarperCollins, 2006.

Fox, Nicols. *It Was Probably Something You Ate.* New York: Penguin Books, 1999.

Korn, Danna. *Kids with Celiac Disease.* Bethesda, Maryland: Woodbine House, 2001.

Lieberman, Shari with Linda Segall. *The Gluten Connection.* Emmaus, Pennsylvania, and New York: Rodale, 2007.

Lord Stewart, Kimberly. *Eating Between the Lines.* New York: St. Martin's Press, 2007.

Sheen, Barbara. *Food Poisoning.* Farmington, Michigan: Lucent Books, 2005.

van Straten, Michael. *Super Feast.* London: Little Books Ltd., 2005.

Vickerstaff Joneja, Janice. *Dealing with Food Allergies in Babies and Children.* Boulder, Colorado: Bull Publishing Company, 2007.

Walsh, William E. *Food Allergies.* New York: John Wiley and Sons, 2000.

Magazines, Journals, and Newspapers

Estruch, Ramon, Miguel Angel Martinez-González, Dolores Corella, et al. "Effects of a Mediterranean-Style Diet on Cardiovascular Risk Factors." *Annals of Internal Medicine* (July 4, 2006) 145: 1–11.

"Ginger and Cancer." *Natural Life* (March–April 2008) 36.

Gorbach, Sherwood L. "Antimicrobial Use in Animal Feed–Time to Stop." *New England Journal of Medicine* (October 18, 2001) 345: 1202–3.

Hobson, Katherine. "'Diets' That Promote Health (and Always Have); Giving Up Their Hunt for Charmed Nutrients, Diet Experts Increasingly Embrace Whole Patterns of Eating." *U. S. News and World Report* (April 7, 2008) NA.

Mitrou, Panagiota N. Victor Kipnis, Anne C. M. Thiébaut, et al. "Mediterranean Dietary Pattern and Prediction of All-Cause Mortality in a US Population." *Annals of Internal Medicine* (December 10/24, 2007) 167: 2461–8.

Rhode, Jennifer, Sarah Fogoros, Suzanna Zick, et al. "Ginger Inhibits Cell Growth and Modulates Angiogenic Factors in Ovarian Cancer Cells." *BMC Complementary and Alternative Medicine* (December 20, 2007) 7: 44.

Sacks, Frank M. "How Safe is Your Food?" *Healthy Eating (Harvard Special Health Report)* (February 2006) 37.

Solan, Matthew. "Healing Foods." *Vegetarian Times* (September 2008) 34: 30–33.

Ward, Elizabeth M. "Suspect Produce: How to Be Safe from Contaminated Fruits, Vegetables." *Environmental Nutrition* (June 2005) 28: 1.

Weinberg, Linda. "A Passion for Produce: Keeping Summer's Bounty Safe to Eat." *Environmental Nutrition* (August 2001) 24: 1.

White, David G., Shaohua Zhao, Robert Sudler, et al. "The Isolation of Antibiotic-Resistant Salmonella from Retail Ground Meats." *New England Journal of Medicine* (October 18, 2001) 345: 1147–54.

Websites

American Heart Association
http://www.americanheart.org

National Foundation for Celiac Awareness
http://www.celiaccentral.org

National Institute of Diabetes and Digestive and Kidney Diseases
http://www2.niddk.nih.gov

National Restaurant Association
http://www.restaurant.org

U.S. Department of Agriculture
http://www.usda.gov
http://www.FoodSafety.gov

Chapter 12

Not Just Cow's Milk

Cow's milk has been a staple of the American diet for generations. Millions of Americans cannot imagine their days without three glasses of milk. Many drink even more. After all, cow's milk contains a host of different nutrients including calcium, protein, vitamins A, D, B12, and K, magnesium, niacin, potassium, and riboflavin. To large numbers of people, cow's milk is one of nature's most complete and perfect foods. According to Stuart Patton, the author of *Milk*, which was published in 2004, "cow's milk contains more of the essential vitamins and minerals required by the human than any other single food."[1] Patton notes a number of different qualities and characteristics of milk that helped to contribute to its "large-scale success." These include the fact that most people like the taste of milk, and "much of the United States is ecologically suited to the pasturing of cattle." In addition, "the physical and chemical properties of milk lend it to transportation and processing in massive volumes."[2]

Furthermore, large numbers of people believe that cow's milk is an essential component of the diet of all non-infant children. Many pediatricians contend that children over the age of one need the nutrients contained in cow's milk, especially the calcium, magnesium, and potassium.

Though cow's milk remains a very popular product, increasing numbers of people are deciding to seek alternative types of milk. There are a number of different reasons for this trend. First, regular cow's milk contains high amounts of fat. The Toronto Vegetarian Association states that even low-fat cow's milk products have high levels of fat. "For example, 2% milk has become much more popular than homogenized milk, yet it still derives one third of its total calories from fat."[3]

In her book, *What to Eat*, which was published in 2006, Marion Nestle, a nutrition professor, explains that dairy foods supply 15 percent of the total fat in the American food supply, "but nearly 30 percent of the

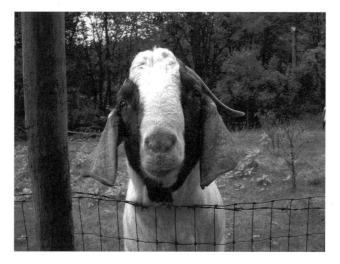

Goats are excellent sources of milk. (Courtesy of Mark A. Goldstein)

saturated fat, the bad kind that raises the risk for heart disease." Furthermore, "nearly 60 percent of the fat in milk is saturated."[4] It is not surprising that Nestle advises her readers to consume milk that has lower levels of fat. To illustrate, she presents the following table:

The Fat and Calories Content of an 8-Ounce Glass of Milk

Milk (percent fat)	Fat (grams)	Saturated Fat (grams)	Calories
Whole (3.25%)	8	5	150
Reduced fat (2%)	5	3	120
Low-fat (1%)	2.5	1.5	100
Nonfat	0.5	0.3	80[5]

In *Cholesterol Cures*, which was written by the editors of *Prevention Health Books* and published in 2002, the authors note that 2 percent milk is not a good option for those who wish to lower their cholesterol levels. "Two percent milk gets 35 percent of its calories from fat, while only 5 percent of the calories in fat-free milk come from fat." Furthermore, people who drink two glasses of 1 percent milk every day for one year, actually consume four pounds of fat. "Drinking the same amount of fat-free milk, on the other hand, provides less than one-tenth of a pound of fat."[6]

Another problem with cow's milk is lactose. Throughout the world, millions of people are unable to digest lactose, the carbohydrate found in cow's milk. They are lactose intolerant. When they drink cow's milk, they may experience a myriad of symptoms such as stomach cramps, diarrhea, and flatulence (gas). Fortunately, once cow's milk is eliminated from the diet (or the lactase enzyme is added to the diet when cow's milk is consumed), people, generally, no longer have these symptoms.

But there is also the problem of the millions of people who have allergies to cow's milk. A 2007 article in *Small Ruminant Research* states that cow's milk contains more than twenty proteins that have the potential to result in allergic reactions. "Hypersensitivity to cow milk proteins is one of the main food allergies and affects mostly but not exclusively infants, while it may also persist through adulthood and can be very severe."[7] Among the symptoms associated with cow's milk allergy are nasal stuffiness, poor appetite, irritability, restlessness, bad breath, hyperactivity, gas, diarrhea, headaches, cramps, constipation, lack of energy, malabsorption of nutrients, runny nose, rashes, eczema, and shortness of breath. The rates of cow's milk allergy appear to be rising. A 2004 article in *Pediatric News* states that "cow's milk protein allergy may be occurring with increased frequency and can even arise in breast-fed infants if the mother consumes enough dairy products." Though the exact rate of cow's milk allergy protein is unknown, estimates range from 0.3 percent to 7 percent.[8]

Still another group that may avoid cow's milk are vegans. (See Chapter 16.) Vegans are vegetarians who also avoid eating dairy products. Obviously, people who have removed dairy products from their diets will not drink cow's milk.

Thankfully, those who no longer consume cow's milk have several alternatives. These include milk obtained from goats, soy, rice, almonds, oats, and hemp.

GOAT MILK

Throughout the world, goat milk is the most popular type of milk. Like cow's milk, goat milk is high in calcium and protein, and goat milk has higher amounts of potassium, chloride, manganese, copper, selenium, niacin, and vitamins B6 and A. (Cow's milk has more vitamin B12 and folic acid than goat milk.) Cow's milk contains eight or nine grams of fat per eight ounces, and goat's milk has ten grams. So it actually has a higher fat content than cow's milk, and it is harder to find low-fat versions of goat's milk than it is to locate those of cow's milk. However, because goat's milk has no agglutinin, the fat globules do not cluster together. As a result, goat milk is easier to digest. Goat's milk also contains more fatty acids that are useful for digestion.

Unlike cow's milk, goat milk has only trace amounts of the allergenic casein protein, alpha-S1, and both cow's milk and goat milk have similar amounts of the allergenic protein, beta-lactoglobulin. Though researchers tend to maintain that children and adults who are allergic to cow's milk will probably be allergic to goat's milk, anecdotal evidence seems to support the opposite. Numbers of people who are allergic to cow's milk appear to be able to tolerate goat milk. As for those who are lactose intolerant, goat's milk has only slightly lower levels of lactose than cow's milk, probably not enough to make a significant difference. Obviously, because goat milk is a dairy product, it is not a suitable alternative for vegans, and similar to other whole or low-fat dairy products, it has cholesterol and saturated fats.

SOYMILK

In the United States, soymilk has become the most popular of all the alternatives to cow's milk. A 2008 article in *Vibrant Life* outlines some of the reasons for its popularity. First, while soymilk contains about the same amount of protein as cow's milk, its protein is derived from soy, a vegetable. "Vegetable proteins are known to generate less calcium loss through the kidneys. Studies confirm that people who get their protein primarily from animal sources are at higher risk for osteoporosis." Second, soymilk has no lactose. That makes soymilk a boost for the millions who are lactose intolerant. Third, soymilk contains high amounts of isoflavones, which are "powerful antioxidants" that are believed to lower the risk for prostate and breast cancer, as well as reduce the discomforts associated with menopause. Isoflavones also lower levels of cholesterol and support bone and heart health. Fortified or enriched forms of soymilk contain vitamins B1, B2, B6, and E, as well as calcium and magnesium.[9]

In *SuperFoods HealthStyle*, which was published in 2006, authors Steven G. Pratt, an ophthalmologist and authority on the role of nutrition and lifestyle in the prevention of disease and optimizing health, and Kathy Matthews extol the merits of all types of soy, including soymilk. "There's no question that soy is a health-promoting food.... The power of soy rests in its benefits as an excellent protein food, its level of essential fatty acids, its supply of vitamins and minerals, its rich supply of fiber, and its health-promoting isoflavones and other phytonutrients."[10] The authors note that the consumption of soy products has been associated with lowering levels of LDL or bad cholesterol; reducing high blood pressure, reducing rates of breast, prostate, and colon cancer; reducing the amount of protein in the urine in people with kidney disease; improved management of diabetes; and lowering risk for osteoporosis.

In an October 2007 interview in *Better Nutrition*, Pratt advises people to substitute soymilk for cow's milk. He suggests that people look for soymilk that is fortified with calcium carbonate instead of tricalcium phosphate, which is more difficult to absorb. And because the calcium tends to settle at the bottom, people should always remember to shake the container.[11]

On the other hand, in the previously noted book *What to Eat*, Nestle says that the research on soy products is far from conclusive. "For every research study in my files that promotes the health benefits of soy foods, I can find another that disputes those benefits." Some studies have even found that soy products cause the problems that it should be correcting. "At the moment, I find it impossible to make sense of the health debates about soy foods, not least because so much of the research is sponsored by industries with a vested interest in its outcome."[12] So what does Nestle advise? Soy products, including soymilk, remain a good substitute for dairy foods and a good source of protein for vegetarians and vegans. "But soy products are not essential, any more than dairy foods are essential." Eating soy foods is simply a matter of personal preference.[13]

A very different opinion is voiced in *The Whole Soy Story*, which was published in 2007, by Kaayla T. Daniel, a nutritionist. Daniel explains that in the United States, soy food products were initially marketed to vegetarians and the poor. However, by the 1970s, to sell soy products to the more affluent, soy was redesigned as "miracle substances that would prevent heart disease and cancer, whisk away flashes, build strong bones and keep us forever young."[14] As a result, soy products are now found in thousands of processed foods. Of course, there is also soymilk.

Although sales of soymilk in 2005 were estimated at around $1 billion, according to Daniel, soymilk is far from a nutritious drink. It "contains pesticide residues along with plant estrogens and other toxins."[15] In fact, Daniel maintains that soy is not a miracle food, the answer to world hunger, or a panacea. It has not even been proven to be safe.[16] And she contends that soy has been linked to the following medical problems: malnutrition, digestive distress, thyroid dysfunction, cognitive decline, reproductive disorders, infertility, birth defects, immune system breakdown, heart disease, and cancer.[17]

There is also the real question of whether children will drink soymilk. In a study published in 2006 in the *Journal of the American Dietetic Association* researchers made both cow's milk and soymilk available to elementary school children. "After four weeks of soymilk availability, 22.3% of students chose soymilk and consumed an average of 58% of each carton, whereas 77.6% chose dairy milk and consumed an average of 52.6%. Total calcium-rich beverage selection with lunch increased from 79% to 83.1%."[18] So it appears, at least from this study, that elementary-age schoolchildren will drink soymilk.

Of course, the jury is still out on soy products. It may be quite some time before there are definitive answers. Still, for the average person, consuming smaller amounts of soymilk is probably not problematic, and those who wish to avoid the pesticides should purchase only organic soy products. An article published in 2006 in *Environmental Health Perspectives* concludes, what most researchers agree on, that we are only just beginning to truly understand the nature of soy and that much more research is needed before it is possible to make firm health recommendations."[19]

RICE MILK

Processed from brown rice, rice milk typically contains a natural sweetener such as rice syrup or evaporated cane juice and is usually fortified with calcium, B12, and/or vitamin D. Unlike cow's milk, which contains protein, fat, and carbohydrates, rice milk is primarily a source of carbohydrates. Because rice milk contains no lactose, it may be consumed by those unable to drink cow's milk. Many brands are also gluten-free. (Some brands convert the brown rice syrup with barley, so they are not gluten-free.) However, a 2008 article in *Vegetarian Journal* underscores the fact that rice milk is not the nutritional equivalent of cow's milk. So it should be seen "as a useful replacement for soymilk or cow's milk for taste and cooking purposes." Those who drink a good deal of rice milk should "eat a wide variety of other foods to insure that you're getting all the nutrients you need."[20]

ALMOND MILK

Although almond milk probably sounds as if it is a relatively new product, it may actually be traced to medieval Europe and even earlier generations in the Middle East. People gravitated toward the high-protein content, and almond milk remained fresher for longer periods of time than dairy products, which tended to sour. Moreover, almonds store easily and, in the thousands of years before refrigeration, they did not require colder temperatures.

Unlike cow's milk, almond milk has no saturated fat, cholesterol, or lactose. It has almost the same amount of protein as cow's milk and is a source of vitamin E, calcium, copper, fiber, iron, magnesium, manganese, phosphorous, potassium, and zinc. Many almond milks are fortified with vitamins A and D. Some also contain higher amounts of additives and sweeteners; it is best to avoid those. The concern about sweeteners is especially important for someone dealing with diabetes and/or excess weight.

In the previously noted 2008 *Vegetarian Journal* article, the author states that "almonds are one of the healthiest nuts that humans can eat." As a result, "almond milk ... may be one of the more nutritious milk alternatives on the market." Yet, because almonds are expensive, there may be only a small amount of almonds in the almond milk.[21] Labels should be read closely.

The American Dietetic Association prepared a "Nutrition Fact Sheet" on almonds. It notes that almonds may play a crucial role in a healthy lifestyle. In fact, they may provide a host of different nutrients and cholesterol-lowering properties without weight gain.[22] Presumably, almond milk that contains a higher percentage of almonds may also have similar benefits.

OAT MILK

Another good options for people who are lactose intolerant or who wish to avoid consuming foods containing animal products is oat milk. Over the years, a number of different studies have found that oats have a myriad of health benefits. For example, research conducted at the American Institute for Cancer Research has found that a diet that includes lots of whole grains, such as oats, lowers the risk of colorectal cancer. Because these foods contain so much fiber, they reduce the amount of time that food moves through the digestive system.[23]

A 2008 article in the *American Journal of Lifestyle Medicine* reviewed the past ten years of oatmeal/cholesterol research. According to the researchers, just about all the studies that have been conducted have found that the "consumption of oats and oat-based products significantly reduces total cholesterol and low-density lipoprotein cholesterol concentrations without adverse effects on high-density liproprotein cholesterol or triglyceride concentrations." Moreover, including oats and oat-based products in the diet "may confer health benefits that extend beyond total cholesterol and low-density lipoprotein cholesterol reduction."[24]

Furthermore, a brief article in a 2000 issue of *Women's Health Letter* cites a small study that was conducted in Sweden. Researchers divided the subjects into two groups. One group drank oat milk for one month and then soymilk for a month. The second group drank oat milk for one month and then cow's milk for the second month. Oak milk was found to lower "cholesterol by four percent and the harmful LDL by nine percent in this short period of time."[25] However, an article that was published a few months later in another issue of *Women's Health Letter* states that some commercial forms of oat milk may contain tricalcium phosphate, which may trigger kidney stones and other calcifications. So labels of commercial forms of oat milk should be read carefully.[26]

HEMP MILK

Before frightening too many people about hemp milk, it is important to note that the leaves and flowering tops of hemp are the parts of the plant that contain THC (tetrahydrocannabinol), the psychoactive chemical found in marijuana. The seeds and nuts portions of the plant, from which hemp milk is made, contain no THC.

While hemp milk has no animal products, it is an excellent source of omega fatty acids, calcium, and phosphorus. It is also high in iron and contains vitamin E, folic acid, niacin, magnesium, thiamin, and zinc. Likewise, hemp milk may be fortified with other vitamins and minerals such as vitamin D, B12, and riboflavin. In *Hemp*, which was published in 2003, author Mark Bourrie explains that, "hemp seeds contain 25 percent high-quality protein and 40 percent fat. Hemp oil has a re-markable fatty acid profile, being high in desirable omega-3 and omega-6 fatty acids and also delivering some GLA (gamma-linolenic acid) that is absent from the fats we normally eat."[27] Inadequate amounts of omega-3 fatty acids may result in inflammatory conditions, heart disease, and skin problems.

A 2007 article in *Prevention* magazine states that hemp is an excellent source of protein. "Hemp seeds are one of the few plant sources of all nine essential amino acids your body needs to build and repair muscle. That's a boon for vegetarians because most nonanimal sources of pro-tein are incomplete."[28]

Hemp milk is a good choice for those worried about the allergens asso-ciated with nuts and soy and for those concerned with environmental issues. When growing hemp, farmers tend to use no herbicides or pesti-cides, and the hemp itself requires little water. And, according to a 2006 ar-ticle in *Better Nutrition*, "unlike much of the soy grown in North America, hemp is never genetically modified, a practice many environmentalists worry will upset our sensitive ecological balance."[29] (It should be noted that it is illegal to grow hemp in the United States. However, since 1998 it has been legal to grow and sell hemp in Canada. The vast majority of the hemp sold in the United States comes from Canada.)

Before concluding, it should be noted that neither cow's milk nor any of the alternative milks should be fed to infants instead of breast milk or infant formula. Apparently, some parents have believed that these products met the nutritional needs of their infants, and their chil-dren developed rickets, as a result of vitamin D deficiency, and kwa-shiorkor, a protein deficiency—problems not seen in the developed world.[30] A 2001 article in *Pediatrics* notes that "these nutritional dis-eases, which are associated with considerable morbidity and possible mortality, are entirely preventable.... The health food beverages used by these families stated on the container that they were not untended for use as infant formulas."[31]

CONCLUSION

While many consider cow's milk to be a near perfect food, for a number of different reasons, it is not an appropriate option for many people. Large numbers of people are either allergic to milk or have lactose intolerance. Some people simply do not wish to consume food that contains animal products.

Thankfully, now there are a host of different options, including goat's milk, soymilk, rice milk, almond milk, oat milk, and hemp milk. Because they are readily available, just about everyone should be able to find a milk that suits his or her needs.

TOPICS FOR DISCUSSION

1. Do you drink regular cow's milk? Are you concerned about the amount of fat it contains? Why or why not?

2. After reading this chapter do you think you will drink lower-fat cow's milk?

   Why or why not?

3. Have you ever had soymilk? Has reading this chapter altered your opinion of soymilk? How?

4. Have you ever consumed any of the alternative milks? Which ones? What were they like?

5. Has reading this chapter changed your consumption of milk? How?

NOTES

1. Stuart Patton, *Milk* (New Brunswick, New Jersey: Transaction Publishers) 1.

2. Stuart Patton, *Milk*, 18.

3. Toronto Vegetarian Association website, http://veg.ca.

4. Marion Nestle, *What to Eat* (New York: North Point Press, 2006) 74.

5. Marion Nestle, *What to Eat*, 76.

6. Editors of *Prevention* Health Books, *Cholesterol Cures* (Emmaus, Pennsylvania, and New York City: Rodale, 2002).

7. E. I. El-Agamy, "The Challenge of Cow Milk Protein Allergy," *Small Ruminant Research* (March 2007) 68: 64–72.

8. Timothy F. Kim, "Cow's Milk Allergy is Being Seen with Increased Frequency," *Pediatric News* (March 2004) 38: 34.

9. Patricia Humphrey, "Milk Alternatives: Are They Safe? Are They Enough? If You're a Vegan, As I Am, I'm Pretty Sure This Topic is of Keen Interest to You. After All, Some 'Health Foods' are Anything But Healthy. Can You Trust Milk Alternatives to Deliver the Nutritional Punch Your Body Needs?" *Vibrant Life* (March—April 2008) 24: 10–11.

10. Steven G. Pratt and Kathy Matthews, *SuperFoods HealthStyle* (New York: William Morrow, 2006) 137.

11. April Girouard, "Soymilk Makes a Splash: Discover What Many Lactose-Intolerant People Already Have—That Soymilk Is a Creamy, Nutritious Alternative to Milk," *Better Nutrition*,(October 2007) 69: 68.

12. Marion Nestle, *What to Eat*, 127–128.

13. Marion Nestle, *What to Eat*, 137.

14. Kaayla T. Daniel, *The Whole Soy Story* (Washington, D.C.: New Trends Publishing, Inc.) 2.

15. Kaayla T. Daniel, *The Whole Soy Story*, 75.

16. The Whole Soy Story website, http://wholesoystory.com.

17. The Whole Soy Story website.

18. Jennifer K. Reilly, Amy J. Lanou, Neal D. Barnard, Kim Seidl, and Amber A. Green, "Acceptability of Soymilk as a Calcium-Rich Beverage in Elementary School Children," *Journal of the American Dietetic Association* (April 2006) 106: 590–593 .

19. Julia R. Barrett, "The Science of Soy: What Do We Really Know?" *Environmental Health Perspectives* (June 2006) 114: A 352–8.

20. Stephanie Gall, "An Updated Guide to Soy, Rice, Nut, and Other Non-Dairy Milks." *Vegetarian Journal* (January—March 2008) 27: 10–16.

21. Stephanie Gall, Stephanie, "An Updated Guide to Soy, Rice, Nut, and Other Non-Dairy Milks," 10–16.

22. "Nutrition Fact Sheet: Almonds: A Handful Can Make a Difference," American Dietetic Association website, http://eatright.org.

23. American Institute for Cancer Research website, http://.aicr.org.

24. Mark B. Andon and James W. Anderson, "State of the Art Reviews: The Oatmeal-Cholesterol Connection: 10 Years Later," *American Journal of Lifestyle Medicine* (February 2008) 2: 51–7.

25. "Lowing Cholesterol Easily," *Women's Health Letter* (October 2000) 6: 7.

26. Nan Kathryn Fuchs, "Check Your Oat Milk," *Women's Health Letter* (December 2000) 6: 7.

27. Mark Bourrie, *Hemp* (Buffalo, New York: Firefly Books, 2003) 71–72.

28. Marge Perry, "The New Health Food Darling," *Prevention* (May 2007) 59: 85.

29. Matthew G. Kadey, "Hemp Does a Body Good; This Superfood Has Nothing to do with Marijuana—And Everything to do with Sound Nutrition and Health," *Better Nutrition* (November 2006) 68: 50–2.

30. Patricia Humphrey, "Milk Alternatives: Are They Safe? Are They Enough? If You're a Vegan, As I Am, I'm Pretty Sure This Topic Is of Keen Interest to You. After All, Some 'Health Foods' are Anything But Healthy. Can You Trust Milk Alternatives to Deliver the Nutritional Punch Your Body Needs?" 10–11.

31. Norman F. Carvalho, Richard D. Kenney, Paul H. Carrington, and David E. Hall. "Severe Nutritional Deficiencies in Toddlers Resulting from Health Food Milk Alternatives," *Pediatrics* (April 2001) 107: 760–1.

REFERENCES AND RESOURCES

Books

Bourrie, Mark. *Hemp*. Buffalo, New York: Firefly Books, 2003.

Daniel, Kaayla T. *The Whole Soy Story*. Washington, D.C.: New Trends Publishing, Inc., 2007.

Editors of *Prevention* Health Books. *Cholesterol Cures*. Emmaus, Pennsylvania, and New York City: Rodale, 2002.

Nestle, Marion. *What to Eat*. New York: North Point Press, 2006.

Patton, Stuart. *Milk.* New Brunswick, New Jersey: Transaction Publishers, 2004.

Pratt, Steven G. and Kathy Matthews. *SuperFoods HealthStyle.* New York: William Morrow, 2006.

Yu, Winnie. *What to Eat for What Ails You.* Gloucester, Massachusetts: Fair Winds Press, 2007.

Magazines, Journals, and Newspapers

Andon, Mark B. and James W. Anderson. "State of the Art Reviews: The Oatmeal-Cholesterol Connection: 10 Years Later." *American Journal of Lifestyle Medicine* (February 2008) 2: 51–7.

Barrett, Julia R. "The Science of Soy: What Do We Really Know?" *Environmental Health Perspectives* (June 2006) 114: A 352–8.

Batz Jr., Bob. "Hemp Milk? It's Health and Legal as Hemp Cereal." Pittsburgh Post-Gazette website, http://www.post-gazette.com.

Carvalho, Norman F., Richard D. Kenney, Paul H. Carrington, and David E. Hall. "Severe Nutritional Deficiencies in Toddlers Resulting from Health Food Milk Alternatives." *Pediatrics* (April 2001) 107: 760–1.

Editors of *Prevention* Health Books. *Cholesterol Cures.* Emmaus and New York: Rodale, 2002.

El-Agamy, E. I. "The Challenge of Cow Milk Protein Allergy." *Small Ruminant Research* (March 2007) 68: 64–72.

Fuchs, Nan Kathryn. *Women's Health Letter* (December 2000) 6: 7.

Gall, Stephanie. "An Updated Guide to Soy, Rice, Nut, and Other Non-Diary Milks."*Vegetarian Journal* (January—March 2008) 27: 10–16.

Girouard, April. "Soymilk Makes a Splash: Discover What Many Lactose-Intolerant People Already Have—That Soymilk is a Creamy, Nutritious Alternative to Milk."*Better Nutrition* (October 2007) 69: 68.

"Goat Milk: Allergen Alternative." *Better Nutrition* (June 2004) 66: 30.

Humphrey, Patricia. "Milk Alternatives: Are They Safe? Are They Enough? If You're a Vegan, As I Am, I'm Pretty Sure This Topic is of Keen Interest to You. After All, Some 'Health Foods' are Anything But Healthy. Can You Trust Milk Alternatives to Deliver the Nutritional Punch Your Body Needs?" *Vibrant Life* (March—April 2008) 24: 10–11.

Kadey, Matthew G. "Hemp Does a Body Good; This Superfood Has Nothing to Do with Marijuana—And Everything to Do with Sound Nutrition and Health." *Better Nutrition* (November 2006) 68: 50–2.

Kim, Timothy F. "Cow's Milk Allergy is Being Seen with Increased Frequency." *Pediatric News* (March 2004) 38: 34.

"Lowing Cholesterol Easily." *Women's Health Letter* (October 2000) 6: 7.

Perry, Marge. "The New Health Food Darling." *Prevention* (May 2007) 59: 85.

Reilly, Jennifer K., Amy J. Lanou, Neal D. Barnard, Kim Seidl, and Amber A. Green. "Acceptability of Soymilk as a Calcium-Rich Beverage in Elementary School Children." *Journal of the American Dietetic Association* (April 2006) 106: 590–3.

Smith, Jacqueline R. "Drink Up and Lather on Goat's Milk: Learn How a Product Widely Consumed in Ancient Greece and Rome is Helping Out Lactose Intolerant and Health Conscious Alike in 'Get Milk.'" *Better Nutrition* (June 2007) 69: 40.

Websites

American Dietetic Association
http://eatright.org

American Institute for Cancer Research
http://www.aicr.org

Center for Science in the Public Interest
http://www.cspinet.org

Pittsburgh Post-Gazette
http://www.post-gazette.com

The Whole Soy Story
http://wholesoystory.com

Toronto Vegetarian Association
http://veg.ca

Chapter 13

Organic Foods

In the supermarket there is a large display of apples that sell for $1.99 per pound. There is also a similar arrangement of organic apples. However, these retail for $2.99 per pound. Are the organic apples worth the extra dollar per pound? Are they healthier than the regular apples?

Until the 1970s there were few commercially available organic foods. Most organic foods were found only at small co-ops. That has all changed. Now organic foods are available at regular suburban grocery stores as well as specialty shops and are purchased by consumers from all Ethnic backgrounds and economic sectors of society. A 2007 article in Brandweek notes that, "Gerber, Hunt's, Orville Redenbacher, Ragu, Swanson and Frito-Lay's Tostitos are but a few of the mainstream players who've crossed to the green side. It also includes big companies that can go green instantly by buying an organic label."[1]

According to the Organic Trade Association, sales of organic foods continue to rise rapidly. Today, organic food sales are at least a sixteen-billion-dollar business. "The fastest-growing food categories and their rates of growth over the previous year are organic meat (55.4 percent), organic sauces and condiments (24.2 percent), and dairy products (23.5 percent)."[2] In *The Way We Eat*, published in 2006, Peter Singer, a philosopher, and Jim Mason, an attorney, wrote, "Organic foods have now made the leap ... to chains like Whole foods, Wild Oats, and Trader Joe's, but also Krogers, Super Target, King Soopers, and Price Chopper. Organic food is now available in about three in four U.S. supermarkets.... The mainstay of the organic movement is still fresh fruit and vegetables, though sales of organic milk, eggs, cheese, and meat are growing rapidly. The range of processed organic food is also expanding and now includes pasta sauces, cereals, corn chips, ice cream, peanut butter, coffee, and even frozen dinners."[3]

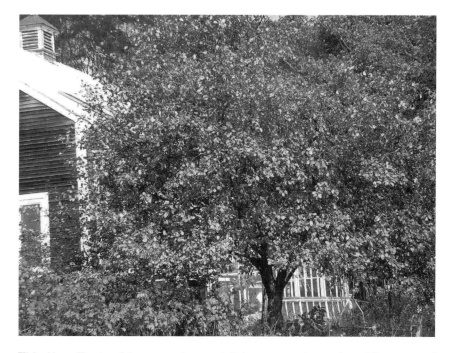

This New England farm produces delicious organic apples. (Courtesy of Mark A. Goldstein)

Who are the consumers who are buying organic foods? An article entitled "Organic Food Strikes Chord with Consumers" that appeared in *MMR: Mass Market Retailers* in 2007 notes that "organic products are moving into the mainstream." A poll conducted by the Hannaford supermarket chain found that "nearly 80% of Hannaford shoppers say they buy organic and natural items at least some of the time." So it seems that large portions of the population are now consumers or potential consumers for organic foods.[4]

STANDARDS FOR ORGANIC FOODS

The United States Department of Agriculture (USDA) notes that "organic food is produced by farms that emphasize the use of renewable resources and the conservation of soil and water to enhance environmental quality for future generations." Foods that are raised organically are fed no antibiotics or growth hormones. "Organic food is produced without using most conventional pesticides; fertilizers made with synthetic ingredients or sewage sludge; bioengineering; or ionizing radiation." Furthermore, before labeling a food "organic," the farm where the food is grown must be inspected by a government-approved certifier. "Companies that handle or process organic food before it gets to your local supermarket or restaurant must be certified, too."[5]

What makes a food organic has little to do with the food; instead, it is primarily a function of how the soil is prepared and how the food is produced. Organic growers manage their farms as whole systems. They focus on improving soil health and use farming methods that prevent problems, such as rotating crops from field to field to manage pests and weeds and to improve soil health and fertility, using animal manures and vegetative matter as fertilizers, monitoring the fields regularly to determine when pest or weed control is needed, and recycling and composting organic waste.

For many years, certification of organic farmers was conducted by more than forty state and private organizations. In December 2000 the USDA issued a universal standard, which became effective in 2002. The standard established four categories for labeling. Foods that are labeled "100 percent organic" must contain only organic ingredients. Ninety-five percent of the ingredients of any food labeled "organic" must be organic. Foods that contain at least 70 percent organic ingredients may contain a label that says, "Made with Organic Ingredients." There are additional restrictions on the remaining 30 percent of ingredients, such as they may not contain any genetically modified organisms (GMOs). "Products with less than 70% organic ingredients may list organically produced ingredients on the side panel of the package, but may not make any organic claims on the front of the package." Organic dairy animals must be fed organic products and have access to the outdoors. In addition, they must not live in crowded conditions.[6]

At the same time, the U.S. Department of Agriculture emphasizes that it "makes no claims that organically produced food is safer or more nutritious than conventionally produced food. Organic food differs from conventionally produced food in the way it is grown, handled and processed."[7]

Two decades ago, the Organic Foods Protection Act (OFPA) of 1990 was passed. It mandated that the USDA create national standards for organically produced agricultural products. To be sold as organic, products needed to adhere to these standards. "The OFPA and the National Organic Program (NOP) regulations require that agricultural products labeled as organic originate from farms or handling operations certified by a State or private entity that has been accredited by USDA. The NOP is a marketing program housed within the USDA Agricultural Marketing Service. Neither the OFPA nor the NOP regulations address food safety or nutrition."[8]

In December 1997, Dan Glickman, who was then the Secretary of Agriculture, suggested that the federal organic standards for U.S. food crops include foods that are genetically engineered and/or irradiated. He also wanted organic farmers to be able to use sewage sludge as fertilizer and confine their livestock. It is not surprising that the Department was inundated with complaints and demands that the rule be rewritten. It is believed that the proposed standards were created following much lobbying from the giant businesses. How else, for example, could one explain the addition of sludge, which contains toxic chemicals and residential, industrial, and commercial discharge? New standards that prohibited the use of genetic engineering and addressed the other contested issues were proposed in March 2000. The standards were further modified, and, as noted, presented in their final form in December 2000.

In *To Buy or Not To Buy Organic,* which was published in 2007, Cindy Burke says that, in an effort to "cut corners," agricultural lobbyists have repeatedly attempted to lower the minimum standards for organic products. "Consumers have been vigilant and beaten back efforts to weaken the standards, but the lobbyists keep trying to allow GMO (genetically modified organism) seeds, sewer sludge, and feedlot conditions to become legal organic standards."[9]

PESTICIDES

Organic farmers use no synthetic pesticides, which are poisonous compounds that are designed to kill elements of nature that damage crops, including insects and fungal pests. As such, they have the potential to cause a variety of medical problems. Information about the effects of pesticides has primarily been obtained from studies of pesticide applicators and farm workers. Common reactions to pesticides include nausea, lung and eye irritation, and temporary nerve damage. Long-term and chronic medical problems have been harder to verify, but farmers using more pesticides seem to be at greater risk than nonfarmers for some forms of cancer and amyotropic lateral sclerosis (Lou Gehrig's disease), and tests on animals indicate that some pesticides may cause birth and immune system defects. It is suspected that many pesticides may interfere with hormonal systems that regulate functions like reproduction. However, no one is really certain if a lifetime of consuming small amounts of pesticides might take a toll on each individual person or the population at large.

In "Organic Agriculture and Food Utilization," which was published in 2007, Kirsten Brandt, a senior lecturer at Newcastle University, United Kingdom, writes, "Studies of workers in the pesticide industry or those using pesticides on farms have indicated increased risk of infertility and Parkinson's disease.... However, studies also showed that, in addition to pesticides, working with copper and other heavy metals such as lead and manganese significantly increased the risk of Parkinson's disease.... So, in countries where copper salts are still allowed in organic farming, organic farmers may not achieve the full reduction in risk for Parkinson's.[10]

In an article published in 2005 in *Earth Island Journal,* investigative journalist Christopher D. Cook writes that each year almost one billion pounds of pesticides are used on crops in the United States, "producing a truly toxic harvest.... Roughly 85 percent of all cropland in America relies on herbicides.... The US accounts for more than one third of the $33.5 billion in global pesticide sales, the vast majority for farming."[11]

Pesticides have been found in air, rain, snow, and fog, and they may easily travel from one location to another. So pesticides used in one area may pass into to a supposedly pesticide-free area. Cook notes that "given just a lazy breeze, toxins can migrate for miles.... Although levels generally diminish, pesticide drift can last for weeks, and sometimes months after application."[12] Even pesticides that have been banned, notes Elaine Marie Lipson in *The Organic Foods Sourcebook,* which was published in 2001, may be found in water and soil for indefinite periods of time.[13]

In "Chemical Trespass: Pesticides in Our Bodies and Corporate Accountability," a report written in 2004 by Kristen S. Schafer, Margaret Reeves, Skip Spitzer, and Susan E. Kegley for the Pesticide Action Network North America, the authors note that ingested pesticides may trigger cancer, wreak havoc with hormones, impede fertility, weaken immune systems, and result in birth defects. "These are just some of the known detrimental effects of particular pesticides at very low levels of exposure. Almost nothing is known about the long-term impacts of multiple chemicals in the body over long periods of time."[14]

The report states that data collected by the U.S. Centers for Disease Control and Prevention (CDC) found that children "are exposed to the highest levels of organophosphorus family of pesticides, which damage the nervous system." In addition, when comparisons were made between different ethnic groups, "Mexican Americans had significantly higher concentrations of five of 17 pesticide metabolites measured in urine."[15]

A 2007 article entitled "Pesticides in Fruits and Vegetables: Are They Harmless—Or Is the Truth That We Don't Really Know?" published in *Choice,* a publication of the Australian Consumers' Association, points to a number of pesticide concerns that consumers should consider. First, there is the question of scientific uncertainty. "It's important to remember that, while science delivers more or less reliable knowledge, there's an element of uncertainty in all research findings. This is of particular concern in studies of pesticide toxicity because the levels allowed in foods are so small that harmful effects may not be immediately obvious." There is also the accumulative effect of different pesticides in the body. "While most experts agree that the risk of cancer from individual pesticides is very low, others are concerned that exposure to a 'cocktail' of pesticides may increase the risk."[16]

The Environmental Working Group (EWG), a nonprofit organization that "uses the power of public information to protect public health and the environment," obtained data from the Department of Agriculture and the Food and Drug Administration on nearly 43,000 tests for pesticides on produce. From this data, the EWG determined that consumers who eat the most contaminated fruits and vegetables are exposed to about 15 pesticides each day; consumers who eat the least contaminated fruits and vegetables are exposed to fewer than two pesticides each day. The following are the most contaminated fruits and vegetables: peaches, apples, sweet bell peppers, celery, nectarines, strawberries, cherries, pears, imported grapes, spinach, lettuce, and potatoes. The following are the least contaminated: onions, avocadoes, sweet corn, pineapples, mango, asparagus, sweet peas, kiwi, bananas, cabbage, broccoli, and papaya.[17]

Because of the prevalence of pesticides, it should not be surprising that there has been a boom in the sales of organic baby food. An article in the April 30, 2007, issue of *Food Institute Report* noted that during the 52 weeks that ended on February 24, 2007, organic baby food sales rose 22 percent to $116 million. During that same period, the sales of all baby foods increased 3.1 percent to $3.7 billion.[18]

Why not simply wash off pesticides? Usually, that is not possible. Some pesticides are not water-soluble. In addition, chemicals may easily penetrate fruits and vegetables. It is possible to peel the fruit or vegetable, but that also peels away valuable nutrients. The wax coating, which is sometimes found on fruits and vegetables, only serves to seal in pesticides. The wax may contain fungicides, coloring agents, and other harmful substances.

Because a number of pesticides break down when they are cooked or processed, it may be advisable to take out the pots and pans and start cooking. Cooking enables the nutrients in certain vegetables, such as carrots and sweet corn, to be better absorbed by the body. In many cases the best option is to include more organic foods in the diet. While organic foods may still have some pesticide residues, they should be in lower levels than conventionally grown produce.

ORGANIC VERSUS CONVENTIONAL

There is evidence that, at least when considering some fruits and vegetables, organic food is healthier than conventional food. In a 2007 study entitled "A Comparative Study of Composition and Post Harvest Performance of Organically and Conventionally Grown Kiwi Fruits," published in *Journal of the Science of Food and Agriculture*, the authors noted that "all the main mineral constituents were more concentrated in organic kiwi fruits, which also have high levels of ascorbic acid and total phenol content, resulting in a higher antioxidant activity."[19]

In "Organic Agriculture and Food Utilization," which was published in 2007, Kirsten Brandt states that, compared with conventional high-input production, organic plant foods tend to have fewer nitrates and less total protein. Moreover, they have a higher proportion of essential amino acids in the protein and higher levels of vitamin C and phytochemicals.[20]

In a 2006 study entitled "Organic Diets Significantly Lower Children's Dietary Exposure to Organophosphorus Pesticides," which was published in *Environmental Health Perspectives*, researchers attempted to determine if children who eat an organic diet are exposed to lower levels of pyrethroid pesticides, a very common type of pesticide. During ten days of the study, the children, who were between the ages of three and eleven, were fed conventional diets; during five days of the study they were fed a diet consisting of organic foods. The children were evaluated through analysis of their saliva and urine. Though the study was small, the findings are interesting. The researchers noted that they "were able to demonstrate that an organic diet provides a dramatic and immediate protective effect against exposures to organophosphorus pesticides that are commonly used in agricultural production [not in households]." They also found that the "children were most likely exposed to these organophosphorus pesticides exclusively through their diet."[21]

Why is this finding so significant? In *Organic Inc.*, which was published in 2007, Samuel Fromartz says that, "At ages one to five, children ... eat three to four times more food per pound of body weight than adults, and their diet is far more concentrated (infants consume seventeen times more apple juice than the U.S. average, for example)." That means that the bodies of children are exposed to proportionally higher amounts of pesticides, and the pesticides may have a stronger impact on their bodies.[22]

BeyondPesticides.org also addresses issues related to children and pesticides. It notes that because the bodies of children are still developing, they are "more sensitive to toxic exposure." There also is now strong evidence that "pesticide exposure can adversely affect a child's neurological, respiratory, immune, and endocrine system, even at low levels. Several pesticides ... are known to cause or exacerbate asthma systems."[23]

In a 2005 article entitled "Acute Illnesses Associated with Pesticide Exposure at Schools," which was published in the *Journal of the American Medical Association*, researchers reviewed data from 2,593 people who developed acute pesticide-related illness from exposure at schools. The researchers concluded that both students and school employees become ill, and they recommended "the implementation of integrated pest management programs in schools, practices to reduce pesticide drift, and adoption of pesticide spray buffer zones around schools."[24]

LIMITATIONS OF ORGANIC FOOD

Organic foods, however, are not necessarily healthful or safe. A high-fat food that is made from organic products remains a food that is high in fat. Likewise, the manure that organic farmers use could contain bacteria. Commenting on the manure, the Organic Trade Association notes that both organic and conventional farmers use manure. It is "part of regular farm soil fertilization programs." However, the certified organic farmers "must have a farm plan detailing the methods used to build soil fertility including the application of manure or composted manure. Certified organic farmers are prohibited from using raw manure for at least 90 days before harvest of crops grown for human consumption."[25]

And, almost always, organically produced food is more expensive than conventionally produced food. The Organic Trade Association says that both organic and conventional foods have many of the same costs, such as costs associated with growing, harvesting, transportation, and storage. But "organically produced foods must meet stricter regulations governing all of these steps, so the process is often more labor- and management-intensive, and farming tends to be on a smaller scale."[26]

ORGANIC FOOD BUSINESS IS GROWING RAPIDLY

Still, there is absolutely no doubt that organic foods are making serious headways in just about every marketplace arena. In a 2006 article in the *Los Angeles Business Journal*, Emily Bryson York describes how the BOA Steakhouse, a "high-end Wilshire Boulevard restaurant," is offering a fourteen-ounce certified organic steak. That means that the steak, which is ruby-red and lower in fat than regular steaks, came from a cow that "grazed on pesticide-free grass and never received any antibiotics or growth hormones."[27] And then there is the cost— $44. In addition to the gamy taste and sinewy texture, the staff at the BOA Steakhouse must deal with a significant problem. "Most people who are really health-conscious don't eat steak."[28]

The organic frozen food business is booming in the United States. In an article that was published in 2007 in *Quick Frozen Foods International*, Mary Davis notes that "a surprisingly large number of companies produce and market frozen food that is organic or contains organic ingredients; and some are still owned by the people who set them up." For example, Davis mentions Amy's Kitchen, which considers itself "the national leading frozen natural foods brand." Founded in 1987, it is still owned by the same family.[29]

Grocery chains, such as Whole Foods, Wild Oats, and Safeway, are even selling their own lines of frozen-organic foods. Davis notes that, "the fact that private label has entered the domain of organics in a big way is a sign that the field is growing.... The range of frozen organic food on the market is enormous. In fact, a consumer could live very well on nothing but organic frozen foods."[30]

Still another area of phenomenal growth is snack food. A 2007 article in *Candy & Snack Business* states that "organic and natural snack sales reached $677 million in 2006, double the amount sold in 2001, and continue to grow."[31] According to this article, about 60 percent of Americans regularly eat snack foods, "receiving about 20% of their calories from snacks." Organic snack bars have been particularly popular. "Snack bar introductions of the organic variety increased 89 percent in 2006 ... versus a 12 percent decline in the conventional segment."[32]

There is even a rising demand for organic pet food. The same people who are buying organic foods for themselves are now beginning to purchase organic pet foods for their dogs and cats. In a 2007 article in *Supermarket News*, Matthew Enis explains that people who purchase organic pet food "tend to fall into a handful of broad groups: foodies, health enthusiasts, avid organic consumers, and empty-nesters." They also want their pets to eat food that is free of antibiotics, hormones, artificial flavors and colors, and rendered animal products.[33]

NOT EVERYONE GRAVITATES TO ORGANICS

As might be anticipated, not everyone believes that organic foods are better than conventional products and worth the extra cost. In a 2007 article entitled "Pesky Organic Pesticides: Dogma Aside, Organic Food Isn't Safer for Us, and It Isn't Better for the Environment" in the *Western Standard*, John Luik maintains that "organic faming uses a range of organic pesticides, about 60 percent of which are know to be rodent carcinogens." Still, he adds, the U.S. Food and Drug Administration's Center for Food Safety and Applied Nutrition has determined that "only about 2.4 percent of domestic foods exceed acceptable pesticide levels."[34]

Moreover, Luik thinks that organic farming is impractical and unrealistic. "Since organic farming is much less intensive, with lower yields, we'd need to devote much more land to farming to produce the same amount of organic food as non-organic." Luik questions whether organic farming could ever produce in sufficient quantities to feed the public.[35]

Nobel Peace Prize winner, Norman Borlaug, an agronomist, expressed similar thoughts in an interview published in 2000 in *Reason*. "Even if you could use all the organic material that you have—the animal manures, the human waste, the plant residues—and get them back on the soil, you couldn't feed more than four billion people. In addition, if all agriculture were organic, you would have to increase cropland area dramatically, spreading out into marginal areas and cutting down millions of acres of forests."[36]

However, a study published in 2007 in *Renewable Agriculture and Food Systems* appears to refute that contention. According to the researchers, organic farming is able to produce a sufficient amount of food to feed the world. From their model estimates they determined that organic methods "could produce enough food supply on a global *per capita* basis to sustain the current human population, and potentially and even larger population, without increasing the agricultural land base." As a result, "organic agriculture has the potential to contribute quite substantially to the global food supply, while reducing the detrimental environmental impact of conventional agriculture."[37]

At the same time, the Center for Global Food Issues maintains that the claims made by these researchers are "not credible" and have the following internal fatal flaws:

- Claiming yields from non-organic farming methods as organic;
- Comparing 'organic' yields to non-representative 'non-organic' yields;
- Double, triple, even quintuple counting of organic yields from the same few research projects;
- Omitting non-favorable crop yields while using favorable yields from the same studies;
- Misreporting yield results.[38]

But how about the quality of the food that is produced on conventional farms? Brian Halwell responds to that concern in a 2007 article entitled, "Still No Free Lunch: Nutrient Levels in U.S. Food Supply Eroded by Pursuit of High Yields," published by The Organic Center. According to Halwell, although farmers now raise two or even three times the amount of food that they raised decades ago, the amounts of nutrients contained in foods has diminished. Thus, "ounce for ounce, today's high-yield crops are less nutritious and deliver fewer nutrients per serving and calories consumed." With so many advances in farming, how could this have happened? "Nutrient decline has occurred because the focus of plant and animal breeders, farmers, and agribusiness has been on increasing yields, not on food nutritional quality."[39]

FOOD QUALITY

In a 2001 article in *Food Processing*, John L. Stanton contests the notion that organic produce is "safer" than conventional produce. In fact, he maintains, since organic food is fertilized with organic matter, it has a higher risk for *E. coli*. In addition, Stanton thinks that free-range chickens have no advantages over those kept in cages. On the contrary, caged chickens are carefully monitored and their intake is controlled. Who knows what the free-range chickens are eating? "Now I am not saying that one is safer than the other. If a consumer feels sorry for chickens that are kept in cages and is willing to pay more to kill and eat a chicken that has run free for a few weeks, so be it—but consumers also believe they are getting a safer product."[40]

In their book, *The Way We Eat*, Peter Singer and Jim Mason explain that the French, British, and Swedish governmental food agencies have stated that there is no proof that organic food is either safer or more nutritious than conventional farmed food. Still, they quote Michael Pollan, who has written about farming for *The New York Times*. According to Singer and Mason, Pollan wrote the following. "The science might still be sketchy, but common sense tells me organic is better food—better, anyway, than the kind grown with organophosphates, with antibiotics and growth hormones, with cadmium and lead and arsenic (the E.P.A. permits the use of toxic waste in fertilizers), with sewage sludge and animal feed made from ground-up bits of other animals as well as their own manure."[41]

PESTICIDES SHOULD BE USED

An article in a 2005 edition of *Farmers Guardian* entitled "Pesticides Crucial to Food Production Future" describes the keynote speech offered by John Pickett at the Pesticides and the Food Chain seminar held in the Rothamsted Research Centre in Hertfordshire, United Kingsom. According to the article, during the speech Professor Pickett said that a combination of factors, including some members of the media and the "malicious practices of pressure groups," are forcing farmers to use very low levels of pesticide residues. This practice has the potential to "result in many existing products being pushed out of the market" and "that would be a disaster for world food supply." Then, Pickett is quoted as follows: "These groups tend to forget that we have to protect our crops against pests, diseases, and weeds ... We cannot possibly provide for our own needs in Europe and those of the world's growing populations if we don't. We have to use something, and, at the moment, that has to be pesticides."[42]

These are essentially the beliefs of Dennis T. Avery, an expert in international agriculture. In *Saving the Planet with Pesticides and Plastic*, which was published in 2000, Avery writes that, given the present level of knowledge about farming, it is unrealistic and impractical, to recommend either the widespread use of organic farming or traditional low-yield farming systems as alternative to high-yield agriculture. "In fact, slashing farm chemical usage is likely to produce more soil erosion, more human cancer, and less wildlife habitat. At present, organic farming could not even sustain the fertility of our existing cropland, or protect it effectively from erosion."[43]

CONCLUSION

Just a few decades ago, organic foods were in short supply. Now, they are found in just about all types of supermarkets—in addition to traditional health food stores. But are organic foods worth the extra cost? Organic foods are produced without the use of synthetic pesticides. People who believe that they may be harmed by consuming small amounts of pesticides and who also have the resources to pay the extra costs associated with organic products will tend to select as many organics as possible. People who believe that pesticides, which have been used for decades, are generally safe or who live on more limited resources, will tend to use conventionally produced products. As this chapter has shown, there is little consensus on the topic.

TOPICS FOR DISCUSSION

1. Do you ever discuss buying organic food products with your family members or friends? If so, what do they say?
2. Do you agree with the four categories of organic labeling? Why or why not? Do you think people take the time to read them carefully? Why or why not?
3. Do you think that ingesting small amounts of pesticides can harm your heath? Why or why not?
4. Do you think it is important for young children to refrain from eating pesticides? Why or why not?
5. Do you think organic foods are healthier than nonorganic foods? Why or why not?

NOTES

1. Kenneth Hein, "The World on a Platter," *Brandweek* (April 23, 2007) 48: 27–8.
2. Organic Trade Association website, http://www.ota.com.
3. Peter Singer and Jim Mason, *The Way We Eat* (New York and Emmaus, Pennsylvania: Rodale, 2006) 197.
4. "Organic Food Strikes Chord with Consumers," *MMR: Mass Market Retailers* (June 18, 2007) 24: 109.
5. U.S. Department of Agriculture website, http://www.usda.gov.
6. National Organic Program website, http://www.ams.usda.gov/nop.
7. U.S. Department of Agriculture website.
8. National Organic Program website.
9. Cindy Burke, *To Buy or Not To Buy Organic* (New York: Marlowe & Company, 2007) 11.

10. Kristen Brandt, "Organic Agriculture and Food Utilization," Author is a senior lecturer at Newcastle University, United Kingdom (May, 2007) 16–17.

11. Christopher D. Cook, "The Spraying of America: American Agriculture Dumps a Billion Pounds of Pesticides on Food, Producing a Truly Toxic Harvest," *Earth Island Journal* (Spring 2005) 20: 34–8.

12. Christopher D. Cook.

13. Elaine Marie Lipson, *The Organic Foods Sourcebook* (Chicago: Contemporary Books, 2001) 13.

14. Pesticide Action Network North America website, http://www.panna.org.

15. Pesticide Action Network North America website.

16. Australian Consumers' Association, "Pesticides in Fruits and Vegetables: Are They Harmless—Or Is the Truth That We Don't Really Know? *Choice* (April 2006) 25–27.

17. Environmental Working Group website, www.ewg.org.

18. "Organic Baby Food Posts Healthy Gains," *Food Institute Report* (April 30, 2007) 8.

19. Maria L. Amodio, Giancarlo Colelli, Janine K. Hasey, and Adel A. Kader, "A Comparative Study of Composition and Post Harvest Performance of Organically and Conventionally Grown Kiwi Fruits," *Journal of Science of Food and Agriculture* (May 2007) 87: 1228–36.

20. Kristen Brandt, 11.

21. Chensheng Lu, Kathryn Toepel, Rene Irish, Richard A. Fenske, Dana B. Barr, and Roberto Bravo. "Organic Diets Significantly Lower Children's Exposure to Organophosphorous Pesticides," *Environmental Health Perspectives* (September 2006) 114: 260–3.

22. Samuel Fromartz, *Organic Inc.* (Orlando, Florida: Harvest, 2007) 3.

23. BeyondPesticides.org website, http://beyondpesticides.org.

24. Walter A. Alarcon, Geoffrey M. Calvert, Jerome M. Blondell, et al., "Acute Illnesses Associated with Pesticide Exposure at Schools," *Journal of the American Medical Association* (July 27, 2005) 294: 455–65.

25. Organic Trade Association website.

26. Organic Trade Association website.

27. Emily Bryson York, "Wholly Cow: Are Trendy Organic Steaks Ready for Prime Time?" *Los Angeles Business Journal* (November 27, 2006) 28: 1–2.

28. Emily Bryson York.

29. Mary Davis, "Organic Frozen Prepared Food in the USA: Still Growing By Leaps and Bounds: Some Small Entrepreneurs that Created the Category Give Way to Big Business As Market Expands, and Major Retailers are Increasingly Getting into the Act with Private Label Offerings," *Quick Frozen Foods International* (January 2007) 48: 103–12.

30. Mary Davis.

31. "Snacks Get a Health Boost: The Organic and Natural Snack Food Segment is Rapidly Expanding and Consumers Become More Aware of What They Eat, Leading to More Variety and Booming Sales," *Candy & Snack Business* (July–August 2007) 18–20.

32. "Snacks Get a Health Boost"

33. Matthew Enis, "Off the Leash: Rising Demand for Organic Meat As Pet Food," *Supermarket News* (March 1, 2007) NA.

34. John Liuk, "Pesky Organic Pesticides: Dogma Aside, Organic Food Isn't Safe for Us, and It Isn't Better for the Environment," *Western Standard* (March 26, 2007) 47–48.

35. John Liuk.

36. Ronald Bailey, "Billions Served" *Reason* (April 2000) 31: 30.

37. Catherine Badgley, Jeremy Moghtader, Eileen Quintero, et al., "Organic Agriculture and the Global Food Supply," *Renewable Agriculture and Food Systems* (July 4, 2007) 22: 86–108.

38. Center for Global Food Issues website, http://www.cgfi.org.

39. The Organic Center website, http://www.organic-center.org.

40. John L. Stanton, "Is Organic Produce Really Safe?" *Food Processing* (June 2001) 52.

41. Singer and Mason, 200–201.

42. "Pesticides Crucial to Food Production Future," *Farmers Guardian* (May 20, 2005) 20.

43. Dennis T. Avery, *Saving the Planet with Pesticides and Plastic* (Indianapolis, Indiana: Hudson Institute, 2000) 171.

REFERENCES AND RESOURCES

Books

Avery, Dennis T. *Saving the Planet with Pesticides and Plastic.* Indianapolis, Indiana: Hudson Institute, 2000.

Burke, Cindy. *To Buy or Not To Buy Organic.* New York: Marlowe & Company, 2007.

Fromartz, Samuel. *Organic Inc.* Orlando, Florida: Harvest, 2007.

Goldsmith, Sheherazade (editor-in-chief). *A Slice of Organic Life.* New York: DK Publishing, 2007.

Lipson, Elaine Marie. *The Organic Foods Sourcebook.* Chicago: Contemporary Books, 2001.

Singer, Peter and Jim Mason. *The Way We Eat.* New York and Emmaus, Pennsylvania: Rodale, 2006.

Magazines, Journals, and Newspapers

Alarcon, Walter A., Geoffrey M. Calvert, Jerome M. Blondell, et al. "Acute Illnesses Associated with Pesticide Exposure at Schools." *Journal of the American Medical Association* (July 27, 2005) 294: 455—65.

Amodio, Maria L., Giancarlo Colelli, Janine K. Hasey, and Adel A. Kader. "A Comparative Study of Composition and Post Harvest Performance of Organically and Conventionally Grown Kiwi Fruits." *Journal of the Science of Food and Agriculture* (May 2007) 87: 1228—36.

Australian Consumers' Association. "Pesticides in Fruits and Vegetables: Are They Harmless—Or Is the Truth That We Don't Really Know?" *Choice* (April 2006) 25–27.

Badgley, Catherine, Jeremy Moghtader, Eileen Quintero, et al. "Organic Agriculture and the Global Food Supply." *Renewable Agriculture and Food Systems* (July 4, 2007) 22: 68–108.

Bailey, Ronald. "Billions Served." *Reason* (April 2000) 31: 30.

Brandt, Kirsten. "Organic Agriculture and Food Utilization," author is a senior lecturer at Newcastle University, United Kingdom (May 2007) 16–17.

Bryson York, Emily. "Wholly Cow: Are Trendy Organic Steaks Ready for Prime Time?" *Los Angeles Business Journal* (November 27, 2006) 28(48): 1–2.

Burke, Cindy. "How to Buy Organic." *Vegetarian Times* (September 2008) 34(8): 52–55.

Cook, Christopher D. "The Spraying of America: American Agriculture Dumps a Billion Pounds of Pesticides on Food, Producing a Truly Toxic Harvest." *Earth Island Journal* (Spring 2005) 20: 34–8.

Davis, Mary. "Organic Frozen Prepared Food in USA: Still Growing By Leaps and Bounds: Some Small Entrepreneurs that Created the Category Give Way to Big Business As Market Expands, and Major Retailers are Increasingly Getting into the Act with Private Label Offerings." *Quick Frozen Foods International* (January 2007) 48: 103–12.

Dell'Amore, Christine B. "Organic Diets Keep Kids Pesticide Free." *UPI Health Business* (February 22, 2006) NA.

Enis, Matthew. "Off the Leash: Rising Demand for Organic Meat As Pet Food." *Supermarket News* (March 1, 2007) NA.

Hein, Kenneth. "The World on a Platter." *Brandweek* (April 23, 2007) 48: 27–8.

Lu, Chensheng, Kathryn Toepel, Rene Irish, Richard A. Fenske, Dana B. Barr, and Roberto Bravo. "Organic Diets Significantly Lower Children's Exposure to Organophosphorus Pesticides." *Environmental Health Perspectives* (September 2006) 114: 260–3.

Luik, John. "Pesky Organic Pesticides: Dogma Aside, Organic Food Isn't Safer for Us, and It Isn't Better for the Environment." *Western Standard* (March 26, 2007) 47–8.

"Organic Baby Food Posts Healthy Gains." *Food Institute Report* (April 30, 2007) 8.

"Organic Food Strikes Chord with Consumers." *MMR: Mass Market Retailers* (June 18, 2007) 24: 109.

"Pesticides Crucial to Food Production Future." *Farmers Guardian* (May 20, 2005) 20.

"Snacks Get a Healthy Boost: The Organic and Natural Snack Food Segment is Rapidly Expanding and Consumers Become More Aware of What They Eat, Leading to More Variety and Booming Sales." *Candy & Snack Business* (July–August 2007) 18–20.

Stanton, John L. "Is Organic Produce Really Safer?" *Food Processing* (June 2001) 52.

Websites

Beyond Pesticides
http://beyondpesticides.org

Center for Global Food Issues
http://www.cgfi.org

Center for the Advancement of Health
http://www.cfah.org

Environmental Working Group
http://www.ewg.org

National Organic Program
http://www.ams.usda.gov/nop

Organic Consumers Association
www.organicconsumers.org

Organic Trade Association
http://www.ota.com

Pesticide Action Network North America
http://www.panna.org

The Organic Center
www.organic-center.org

United States Department of Agriculture
http://www.usda.gov

Chapter 14

Popular Diets

Vast numbers of Americans are overweight. In many ways, obesity is a national epidemic. So it should not surprise anyone that a host of different diets are available. Some seem to be quite helpful, though their long-term effects are unclear.

According to the Weight-control Information Network at the National Institute of Diabetes and Digestive and Kidney Diseases (NIDDK) approximately two-thirds of adults in the United States are overweight; almost one-third are obese. That means that about 133.6 million adult men and women are either overweight or obese. Of these, 68.3 million are men, and 65 million are women.[1] A normal body-mass index (BMI) is between 18 and 24. People with a BMI of 25 are viewed as overweight; those with a BMI of 30 or higher are obese. To calculate BMI, multiply weight in pounds by 703. That number should be divided by the height in inches. Finally, divide the number a second time by the height in inches.

The high rates of excess weight exact a terrible toll on individuals and society at large. Overweight and obese people are at far greater risk for a host of medical problems, such as heart disease, stroke, gallbladder disease, type 2 diabetes, osteoarthritis, high blood pressure, sleep apnea, high blood cholesterol, and certain types of cancer (breast, colorectal, endometrial, and kidney). Obesity has also been associated with complications of pregnancy, menstrual irregularities, hirsutism (excess body and facial hair), stress incontinence (urine leakage), psychological disorders such as depression, increased surgical risk, and increased mortality.[2] Furthermore, society simply favors thinner people. Just look at the most sought-after movie and television stars. Think about the famous people and models on the covers of magazines. There are very few who are overweight or obese. They gain notoriety in part because they stand out from the crowd.

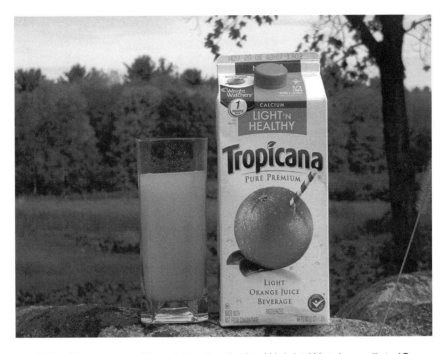

Each food has a specific point value in the Weight Watchers diet. (Courtesy of Mark A. Goldstein)

The numbers of overweight and obese children and teens are also on the rise. In the United States today, obesity in children and teens is reaching epidemic proportions. In a survey conducted between 1976 and 1980, the Centers for Disease Control and Prevention found about 5 percent children between the ages of two and five were overweight. By 2003 to 2004, that figure had grown to 13.9 percent. Meanwhile, in children between the ages of six and eleven, the figure rose from 6.5 percent to 18.8 percent. In teens from the ages of twelve to nineteen, the figure went from 5 percent to 17.4 percent.[3] African-American and Mexican-American children and teens are becoming heavier than their white counterparts. It is believed that cultural factors are playing a role. Pima, Navajo, and Cherokee American children and teens also have even higher rates of excessive weight. A 2006 article in *Harvard Health Commentaries* notes that overweight children are at increased risk for developing cardiovascular problems such as high cholesterol and high blood pressure. In addition, "overweight children are at greater risk for bone and joint problems, sleep apnea, and social and psychological problems such as stigmatization and poor self-esteem."[4] Today's kids are less active than past generations; in an attempt to save money, many schools have eliminated physical recreation. They also spend lots of time watching television, sitting at the computer, and playing video games and are more likely to eat empty-calories foods or foods with higher calories that have little or no nutritional value. Because overweight and obese Children are likely to become overweight adults, they may have the previously noted medical problems associated with overweight and obese adults.

Clearly, genetics and family eating patterns play a role in weight gain. Children who are overweight usually have at least one parent who is overweight. It is not uncommon for every member of the family to be overweight.

Yet the United States is a country obsessed with weight loss. If one types the word "diet" in one of the larger Internet bookstores, hundreds of selections appear. It is not an exaggeration to say that every year people in the United States spend billions of dollars on weight loss. The nonprofit Calorie Control Council estimates that in 2007, 29 percent of the U.S. population was on some type of weight-loss diet. But even after they lose weight, the vast majority of people regain it— some regain more than they lost. While no chapter is able to cover all of the diet approaches that have gained prominence, it is useful to review a few of the most common ones.

WEIGHT WATCHERS

For most of her life, Sarah Ferguson, the ex-wife of Prince Andrew of England, battled excess weight. Over and over again, the duchess tried to lose pounds. After her marriage ended in the mid-1990s, Weight Watchers International asked her to be a spokesperson. She was startled by the offer. "Here I was, a single working mother who certainly had her share of highs and lows in life as well as with my weight. How could I motivate others to take control of their lives when I was still struggling with mine?"[5]

Nevertheless, Sarah accepted the challenge. Sure enough, she lost a good deal of weight. More than a decade later, she remains slim and quite attractive. She is now a Lifetime member and continues to work with the company.

In the past, Weight Watchers offered only one plan. The Flex Plan is a point system based on calories, fat, and fiber. Each food had a specific point value. People consume a set number of points each day; they keep a careful tally of the point values of foods consumed. Obviously, foods with higher point values must be eaten in moderation, but nothing is off limits. The diet tends to be lower in calories and high in fiber.

There is now a second plan, known as the Core Plan. According to Weight Watchers International, it contains foods that are low in energy density. They have fewer calories per ounce. "That means they'll make you feel more satisfied while you are actually consuming fewer calories. You can mix and match these foods as much as you want, and you'll learn to stay aware of hunger and fullness, so you won't overeat."[6] Core Foods include brown rice, lean meats, potatoes, and avocados. "Along with eating any Core Foods you want, you get a 'Weekly Allowance' for foods that aren't on the Core Plan. You can use them for treats, a night on the town, or a special occasion—so you can still indulge sometimes, without going off track."[7]

A key component of the Weight Watchers strategy is support. People who follow this diet may attend weekly meetings led by program graduates. During the meetings, dieters have confidential weigh-ins, share helpful strategies, and obtain expert advice. Weight Watchers maintains that, "Support can be an important part of your weight loss success. In fact, in a study of women trying to lose weight, getting support accompanied an improvement in the participants' ability to control their eating and choose lower-calorie foods." Each week, about 1.5 million people attend meetings throughout the world.[8] When a number of employees want to follow the program at the same time, Weight Watchers will even set up meetings at work-site locations.

However, people who do not have the time or desire to attend meetings may follow their progress online. "We know you have a busy life, and Weight Watchers Online makes it easy to stay connected anywhere, anytime. It's built on the proven approach to weight loss developed by the experts at Weight Watchers—it's practical, liveable, and sustainable."[9]

The Weight Watchers diet has been generally well received. It does require a good deal of vigilance and patience. But there are no foods to weigh or calories to count. One does not need to scrutinize labels or purchase Weight Watchers products.

Weight Watchers does not promise quick weight loss. Though some dieters lose up to two pounds a week, the Weight Watchers program is premised on slow, steady progress and lifestyle changes. Once weight loss is achieved, one remains on a maintenance program. Self-conscious men might think twice before joining. Because Weight Watchers meetings are composed almost entirely of women, they may prefer to join Weight Watchers Online for Men.

THE BEST LIFE

Created by Bob Greene, an exercise physiologist and certified personal trainer, and endorsed by Oprah, The Best Life is a three-phrase program that is more a "way of living" than a diet. The goal is to achieve optimum health.[10]

During Phase One of the program, which lasts for at least four weeks, the focus is on increasing levels of activity and changing meal patterns. Upon beginning the program, people should weigh themselves but then refrain from weighing for at least four weeks. Eat three nutritious meals each day and one snack. Drink plenty of water and eliminate alcoholic drinks (they may be added later). There is no eating for at least two hours before bedtime. And add supplementation. In Bob Greene's book, *The Best Life Diet*, which was published in 2006, he recommends taking a daily multivitamin and mineral supplement as well as an omega-3 fatty acid supplement and, possibly, calcium. For smokers or those on birth control pills, taking extra vitamin C is a good idea.[11]

During Phase Two of the program, Greene deals with the notion of emotional eating. People are told to delve deeper into their emotions and determine why they overeat. It is also important to understand the physical nature of hunger. "One of the benefits of eating regular meals and snacks is that you address your hunger before you get to the point of feeling famished and overeating."[12] Moreover, this phase is the time to practice portion control and remove six "empty calorie," foods, such as soda, from your diet. Phase Three offers lifestyle suggestions, such as meal ideas and fitness plans.

Before beginning this program, be aware of one important issue. There are a number of foods that have received a "Best of Life" seal of approval from Greene. People may easily follow this diet plan without purchasing any of these foods.

HIGH-PROTEIN DIETS

Some people believe that the solution to weight loss lies in high-protein diets or diets that include a higher proportion of protein than most people consume. They argue that this is how humans are genetically programmed to eat.

Clearly, protein is a vital component of everyone's diet. It is an important nutrient for growing, maintaining, and repairing cells. Without protein, the body is unable to regulate fluids, and the immune system cannot function. Protein is required to produce hormones and enzymes. Protein builds skin, bones, and muscle. Our bodies are formed from the protein we obtain from foods.

There are a number of different types of high-protein diets. A 2006 *Harvard Health Commentaries* article notes that high-protein diets range from the "literal Atkins diet as prescribed, to the eating pattern recommended for diabetics, who need to be especially careful about foods that affect blood sugar (primarily carbohydrates). Other choices include Protein Power, Sugarbusters, The Zone, and the many variations of these specific plans that people adapt for themselves in the process of making a diet work for them."[13]

This same article states that the primary advantage of a high-protein diet is that it reduces the consumption of refined carbohydrates, such as white bread, white rice, soda, sweets, and jams and jellies. So, there is better control of blood sugar levels and a reduction in weight and blood-triglyceride levels. But a high-protein diet also lowers the intake of the healthier carbohydrates found in whole grains, as well as fruits and vegetables.

The article further says that Harvard researchers have determined that satisfaction with a weight loss program "is a key factor in successful weight loss." People on high-protein diets that include some high fat content tend to be more satisfied with eating smaller amounts of food.[14]

An article published in 2006 in *Science News* describes research at the University College London in which normal-weight and obese people were injected with the hormone peptide YY (PYY), which is secreted into the gut during and after a meal. Both groups of people reduced their food intake by about one-third. Having obtained these results, the researchers wanted to determine if the amount of secreted PYY varies according to the amounts of protein, carbohydrates, and fats. Normal-weight and obese men were recruited. "The researchers found that blood concentrations of PYY were significantly higher in both groups of men after the high-protein meal than after meals high in carbohydrates or fat. Both groups reported higher sensations of full-ness and less hunger after eating more protein."[15]

Another article on the same research, published in 2006 in *Neutraceuticals International*, notes that the lead researcher "estimates that only slight changes in our diet could go a long way in controlling our weight. She says that a 2 to 3 percent increase in protein consumption and small reductions in carbohydrate consumption might be all that is required to help people lose weight."[16]

But while acknowledging the efficacy of high-protein diets, many health providers have questioned their safety. In fact, there are organizations that have taken a stand against high-protein diets. One of these is the American Heart Association: "Most of these diets aren't balanced in terms of the essential nutrients our bodies need. Some are high in protein and emphasize foods like meat, eggs and cheese, which are rich in protein and saturated fat. Some restrict important carbohydrates such as cereals, grains, fruits, vegetables and low-fat dairy products. If followed for a long time, they can result in potential health problems."[17]

The American Heart Association also states that eating too many foods that are high in fat places people at increased risk for coronary artery disease, diabetes, stroke, and several types of cancer. In addition, people who have bodies that cannot process excess amounts of protein may be at increased risk for kidney and liver disorders.[18]

As might be expected, not everyone agrees with the American Heart Association. In an article published in 2004 in the *Journal of the International Society of Sports Nutrition*, the author says that there is little evidence to support the notion that a high-protein diet negatively impacts liver function or harms healthy kidneys. Furthermore, "a negative correlation has been shown between protein intake and systolic and diastolic blood pressure in several epidemiological surveys." The author stresses that, "for individuals with normal renal function, the risk is minimal and must be balanced against the real and established risk of continued obesity."[19]

Still, an article in 2007 in the *Journal of the American Dietetic Association* reminds those with chronic kidney disease to avoid high-protein diets, which may "accelerate renal deterioration." Moreover, while there is only limited information on the topic, "it appears that high intake of animal and vegetable proteins accelerates the underlying disease process not only in physiologic studies but also in short-term interventional trials."[20]

YOU ON A DIET

Physicians Michael F. Roizen and Mehmet C. Oz have become well-known for their books and appearances on *Oprah*. So it is not surprising that their *You on a Diet*, which was published in 2006, has become a bestseller.

The authors contend that people who want to lose weight should have more knowledge about the digestive process and the "biology of fat."

Here's how the system starts: Before a morsel even reaches the tollbooth, your body has a radar gun to let you know that food is coming—powered by such physiological cues as sight, smell, and the fact that you've been drooling like an overheated Saint Bernard at the thought of a fried-cheese appetizer special. In response to that sensory information, glands in your mouth start to secrete enzymes to help break down your food; then your stomach quickly constructs its version of a roadside welcome center by pumping out stomach acid to help prepare your body for the digestion process.[21]

The actual diet consists of a "fourteen-day rebooting program." Each day, while eating three meals and two snacks, dieters consume about 1,700 calories. Dessert is permitted every other day. Dieters are encouraged to focus on eating whole grains, nuts, lean meats, vegetables, fruits, and fish; they are strongly discouraged from consuming saturated fats, trans fats, and foods that contain high amounts of high-fructose corn syrup. As for beverages, water, seltzer, skim milk and tea are permitted. Up to two diet sodas and up to eight ounces of fruit or vegetables juice fortified with calcium and vitamin D are also allowed. Dieters may drink one alcoholic beverage, and all eating must stop by 8:30 p.m.

Because exercise is an essential part of good health as well as weight loss, the authors recommend thirty minutes of walking and stretching each day. In addition, three days a week, dieters should make time for a twenty-minute strength training routine. For these, the book contains easy-to-follow illustrations. There are even chapters that discuss the roles that hormones and emotions play in overeating.

While Elisa Zied, a spokesperson for the American Dietetic Association, has mostly praise for this diet, she maintains that it has a few problematic areas. First, the diet deemphasizes calorie counting. "Paying attention to approximately how many calories one consumes can be a useful strategy for those trying to lose weight and keep it off, especially at the beginning of any attempt to modify food intake."[22]

Furthermore, Zied says that the recommended menus contain few low-fat dairy foods or other sources of calcium, "which can make it tough for many to meet their calcium and vitamin D needs without supplementation." And Zied believes that the diet includes many foods not commonly eaten in the United States, which makes "the program a challenge over the long term." Still, Zied says that the book is "warm, witty and encouraging," and it may well help "promote both weight loss and improved overall health."[23]

VOLUMETRICS

Developed by Barbara Rolls, a professor at Pennsylvania State University, volumetrics teaches people to eat foods that weigh the same but have fewer calories. So, dieters replace foods that have lots of calories for their weight, such as ice cream and cake, with foods that have lots of bulk, such as fruits, vegetables, and whole grains. The goal is to feel comfortably full with fewer calories. In her book, *The Volumetrics Eating Plan*, which was first published in 2005 and published in trade paper in 2007, Rolls outlines the key principles of volumetrics:

Volumetrics

- focuses on what you can eat, not on what you must give up
- is based on sound nutritional advice widely accepted by health professionals
- emphasizes that the only proven way to lose weight is to eat fewer calories than your body uses as fuel for your activities
- stresses that when you are managing calories it is more important than ever to eat a good balance of foods and nutrients
- teaches you to make food choices that will help control hunger and enhance satiety
- shows you how to fit your favorite foods into your diet
- reinforces eating and activity patterns that you can sustain for a lifetime of achieving your own healthy weight[24]

So to drop the pounds, people should concentrate on eating foods that are less dense or foods with lots of fiber and water. Thus, for example, a 2005 article in *U. S. News & World Report* notes, "pasta, which absorbs water as it cooks, is about half as energy dense as Italian bread, even though the ingredients are similar. Adding water or water-rich foods, like vegetables, and using oils and energy-dense ingredients sparingly lower the density of most dishes, allowing larger portions and increasing satiety."[25]

Volumetrics also stresses the importance of exercise. Rolls says that exercise burns calories "during exercise, but also keeps burning them at a high rate for several hours after you exercise." Exercise builds muscle and reinforces a commitment to a "healthier lifestyle."[26]

OTHER POPULAR DIETS

The following is a listing of still more popular diets:

The UltraSimple Diet, The Fat Smash Diet, The No S Diet, From Belly Fat to Belly Flat Diet, The South Beach Diet, The Best Diet Solution, The Abs Diet, Flat Belly Diet, Jenny Craig, The Hot Latin Diet, Perricone Prescription, Life Choice, macrobiotic, raw foods, Mediterranean Diet, Slim Fast, Glycemic Impact Diet, NutriSystem, Medifast Diet, Bible Based Diet, Dr. Phil Weight Loss Challenge, Eat for Life, The Biggest Loser, Real Age Diet, and Andrew Weil: Eating Well for Optimum Health.

ESSENTIAL DIET PRINCIPLES

If people want to lose weight and maintain the weight loss, which diet should they follow? That is not always clear. In all probability people who adhere to any of the previously discussed diet will initially lose weight. Between the food restrictions and the caloric limitations, the pounds are bound to fall. When people return to their pre-diet eating patterns and find excuses not to exercise, they will regain weight. That is why many health providers advise their patients to make long-term, healthy dietary changes that are combined with lifestyle modifications. While it is evident that there is no one diet that meets the needs of everyone, there are essential principles that will help most people maintain a healthier weight.

In *The American Dietetic Association Complete Food and Nutrition Guide*, third edition, which was published in 2006, Roberta Larson Duyff lists a number of basic ADA dietary guidelines. The goal is to present a sensible, easy-to-follow diet that may readily fit into the average person's lifestyle, rather than a fad diet that one rigorously follows for a period of time, before quitting in abject frustration. People should eat a variety of foods and participate in some form of physical activity. Diets should contain lots of grain products, vegetables, and fruit. They should include a little healthier fat (see chapter 4) but should have little or no saturated fat and no trans fat. Only modest amounts of sugar and salt should be used. If alcohol is consumed, it should be limited. "Different food groups—and the nutrients and other substances their foods provide—help keep you healthy in different ways. No one nutrient, food, or food group has all you need, and none works alone. Health benefits come when your overall eating plan is varied and healthful, without excessive calories."[27]

People should cook with small amounts of monounsaturated fats and watch for hidden fats, especially trans fats, in processed foods. They should consume more foods with fiber. Insoluble fibers, such as wheat bran, aid in digestion; soluble fibers, such as oat bran, seem to help lower cholesterol and regulate the body's use of sugars. In addition, because foods with fiber make the body feel fuller, people who eat them are able to eat less and better control their weight.

The American Heart Association adds that many Americans could lose weight if they controlled their intake of calories and exercised more. In *American Heart Association Low-Fat Low-Cholesterol Cookbook*, third edition, which was published in 2004, the AHA suggests "30 to 60 minutes of moderate exercise on most days of the week. Even moderate levels of regular low-intensity physical activity, such as walking, dancing, and housework, are beneficial."[28]

In *Cleveland Clinic Healthy Heart Lifestyle Guide and Cookbook*, which was published in 2007, the authors contend that weight management is essentially a function of basic mathematics. "If the amount of calories you consume from food equals the number your body metabolizes or 'burns off' from activity, you will maintain your weight. If you consume fewer calories than your body needs for metabolism and activity, you will lose weight. And, in most cases, if you consume more calories than your body needs for these metabolic processes, you will gain weight."[29]

CONCLUSION

The 1.3 million people who live in Okinawa, a chain of islands that stretches from Japan to Taiwan, have one of the longest life expectancy rates in the world. Not only do Okinawans live longer, they are far healthier, and they tend to be slim.

What about their lifestyle lends itself to good health and long life? About three-quarters of their diet is from plants. Every day, they eat between nine and seventeen servings of vegetables and between seven and thirteen servings of whole grains. There are ample amounts of foods with antioxidants and calcium and relatively low amounts of fat, refined sugars, and protein. Furthermore, they practice a cultural habit called "hara hachi bu," in which they stop eating when they feel the first hint of fullness. Exercise is woven into everyday life. "Okinawans keep fit in all three components of fitness—anaerobic, flexibility, and aerobic—mainly through martial arts, which they have been practicing for centuries; traditional dance, which many Okinawan men and women learn from a very young age and continue to perform; and gardening and walking."[30]

Perhaps, instead of gravitating to one of the popular diets, Americans might do better to model their diets and aspects of their lifestyle after the Okinawans, with moderation in both eating habits and exercise. By eating reasonable amounts of more plant-based foods and including regular exercise in their lifestyles, greater numbers of Americans could drop the pounds and improve their health in a safe and sensible way.

TOPICS FOR DISCUSSION

1. Are you overweight? If so, do you have any related medical problems? What are you doing about the situation?

2. Have you heard about any of the diets listed? Have you tried any of them? Describe your experience.

3. Briefly outline your daily diet. What changes do you think you should make? Why?

4. Is exercise a regular part of your life? Why or why not?

5. What do you think people should do to maintain a healthy weight? What changes are you making? Why?

NOTES

1. Weight-control Information Network, National Institute of Diabetes and Digestive and Kidney Diseases website, http://win.niddk.nih.gov.

2. Weight-control Information Network, National Institute of Diabetes and Digestive and Kidney Diseases website.

3. Centers for Disease Control and Prevention website, http://www.cdc.gov.

4. "Food for Thought: How Can We Help Our Kids?" *Harvard Health Commentaries* (August 21, 2006) NA.

5. Mountbatten-Windsor, Sarah, Duchess of York, and Weight Watchers, *Dieting with the Duchess* (New York: Simon and Schuster, 1998) 11.

6. Weight Watchers International website, http://www.weightwatchers.com.

7. Weight Watchers International website.

8. Weight Watchers International website.

9. Weight Watchers International website.

10. The Best Life website, www.thebestlife.com.

11. Bob Greene, *The Best Life Diet* (New York: Simon & Schuster, 2006) 63.

12. Bob Greene, *The Best Life Diet*, 70.

13. "Low-Carb, High-Protein Diets." *Harvard Health Commentaries* (August 21, 2006) NA.

14. "Low-Carb, High-Protein Diets," NA.

15. "High-Protein Diets Boost Hunger-Taming Hormone," *Science News* (September 9, 2006) 173.

16. "European Scientists Unveil Evidence that High-Protein can Lead to Weight Loss," *Neutraceuticals International* (October 2006) NA.

17. American Heart Association website, http://www.americanheart.org.

18. American Heart Association website.

19. Anssi H. Manninen, "High-Protein Weight Loss Diets and Purported Adverse Effects: Where is the Evidence?" *Journal of the International Society of Sports Nutrition* (May 10, 2004) 1: 45–51.

20. Adam Bernstein, Leo Treyzon, and Zhaoping Li, "Are High-Protein Vegetable-Based Diets Safe for Kidney Function? A Review of the Literature," *Journal of the American Dietetic Association* (April 2007) 107: 644–50.

21. Michael F. Roizen and Mehmet C. Oz, *You on a Diet* (New York: Free Press, 2006) 54.

22. American Dietetic Association website, http://eatright.org.

23. American Dietetic Association website.

24. Barbara Rolls, *The Volumetrics Eating Plan* (New York: Harper, 2007) 3.

25. Amanda Spake, "Eat More Weigh Less," *U. S. News & World Report* (March 7, 2005) 138: 50.

26. Barbara Rolls, *The Volumetrics Eating Plan*, 44.

27. Roberta Larson Duyff, *American Dietetic Association Complete Food and Nutrition Guide*, 3rd ed. (Hoboken, New Jersey: John Wiley & Sons, Inc., 2006) 8.

28. *American Heart Association Low-Fat, Low-Cholesterol Cookbook*, 3rd ed. (New York: Clarkson Potter, 2004) 13.

29. Bonnie Sanders Polin and Frances Towner Giedt, *Cleveland Clinic Healthy Heart Lifestyle Guide and Cookbook* (New York: Broadway Books, 2007) 12.

30. Bradley J. Willcox, D. Craig Willcox, and Makoto Suzuki, *The Okinawa Program* (New York: Clarkson Potter, 2001) 7.

REFERENCES AND RESOURCES

Books

American Heart Association Low-Fat Low-Cholesterol Cookbook, 3rd ed. New York: Clarkson Potter, 2004.

Duyff, Roberta Larson. *American Dietetic Association Complete Food and Nutrition Guide*, 3rd ed. Hoboken, New Jersey: John Wiley & Sons, Inc., 2006.

Greene, Bob. *The Best Life Diet.* New York: Simon & Schuster, 2006.

Mountbatten-Windsor, Sarah, Duchess of York, and Weight Watchers. *Dieting with the Duchess.* New York: Simon and Schuster, 1998.

Polin, Bonnie Sanders and Frances Towner Giedt. *Cleveland Clinic Healthy Heart Lifestyle Guide and Cookbook.* New York: Broadway Books, 2007.

Roizen, Michael F. and Mehmet C. Oz. *You on a Diet.* New York: Free Press, 2006.

Rolls, Barbara. *The Volumetrics Eating Plan.* New York: Harper, 2007.

Willcox, Bradley J., D. Craig Willcox, and Makoto Suzuki. *The Okinawa Program.* New York: Clarkson Potter, 2001.

Magazines, Journals, and Newspapers

Bernstein, Adam, Leo Treyzon, and Zhaoping Li. "Are High-Protein, Vegetable-Based Diets Safe for Kidney Function? A Review of the Literature." *Journal of the American Dietetic Association* (April 2007) 107: 644–50.

"European Scientists Unveil Evidence that High-Protein can Lead to Weight Loss." *Nutraceuticals International* (October 2006) NA.

"Food for Thought: How Can We Help Our Kids?" *Harvard Health Commentaries* (August 21, 2006) NA.

"High-Protein Diets Boost Hunger-Taming Hormone." *Science News* (September 9, 2006) 170: 173.

"How to Feel Full on Fewer Calories—For Real." *Tufts University Health & Nutrition Letter* (February 2000) 17: 8.

Lindsay, Jane. "Higher Treatment Costs Associated with Obese Kids." *DOC News* May 2007: 21.

"Low-Carb, High-Protein Diets." *Harvard Health Commentaries* (August 21, 2006) NA.

Manninen, Anssi H. "High-Protein Weight Loss Diets and Purported Adverse Effects: Where Is the Evidence?" *Journal of the International Society of Sports Nutrition* (May 10, 2004) 1: 45–51.

Spake, Amanda. "Eat More Weigh Less." *U. S. News & World Report* (March 7, 2005) 138: 50.

Websites

American Dietetic Association
http://eatright.org

American Heart Association
http://www.americanheart.org

The Best Life
www.thebestlife.com

Calorie Control Council
http://www.caloriecontrol.org

Centers for Disease Control and Prevention
http://www.cdc/gov

National Health Information Center
healthfinder.gov

Weight-control Information Network
National Institute of Diabetes and Digestive and Kidney Diseases (NIDDK)
http://win.niddk.nih.gov

Weight Watchers International
http://weightwatchers.com

Chapter 15

Raw Food

Imagine a kitchen without an oven. No need for a toaster, pots and pans, or a microwave. Instead, the kitchen contains a blender, seed or nut mill, citrus juicer, food hydrator, food processor, sprouting equipment, and colanders.

Visualize a day beginning without a hearty breakfast. No scrambled eggs, no cereal, no bacon, not even a few pieces of toast. In the place of those foods, there is a large bowl of fruit and a hand-full of nuts. Nothing has been cooked. Who eats this type of diet? They are raw foodists or people who eat a raw food diet. Because they avoid using heat to prepare their food, they do not bake, steam, fry, sauté, boil, microwave, or pasteurize their food.

Raw foodists say that raw foods are nutritionally complete. Not only is cooking food unnatural but it actually harms the food. According to raw foodists, when food is cooked, enzymes that are so critical to the digestive process, are killed. A 2003 article in *The Seattle Times* notes that raw foodists "believe that cooking destroys their natural enzymes and depletes their nutritional value. Some contend that foods should never be heated beyond 118 degrees, the temperature at which raw foodists say healthy enzymes start to break down...."[1] (The American Dietetic Association disagrees with this concept. It maintains that the body produces the enzymes needed to digest and absorb food, and any enzymes contained in foods are inactivated by the acids in the stomach.[2])

In her 2004 book *Rawsome!* Brigitte Mars notes that "enzymes exist in all living things and in each of our cells. In fact, enzymes are the 'living sparks' needed for every chemical action and reaction in the body. Over 3,000 enzymes have so far been identified, and researchers believe that many thousands more have yet to be discovered."[3]

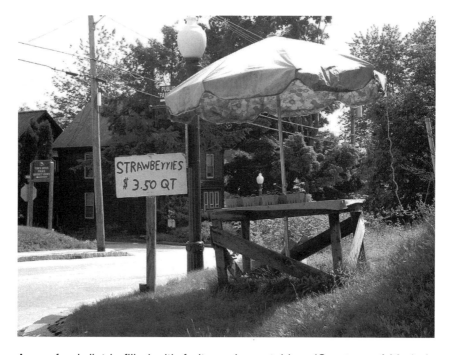

A raw food diet is filled with fruits and vegetables. (Courtesy of Mark A. Goldstein)

Adhering to a raw food diet is not a new concept. Raw foodists say that our early ancestors did not cook their food and that "we didn't evolve to eat cooked food." Moreover, raw foodists note that no other creature on the planet cooks his or her food. Furthermore, cooked food is "at odds with our genetic make-up."[4] In his book, *The Raw Foods Resource Guide,* Jeremy Safron writes, "In the beginning, all creatures consumed their food in a raw form. Somewhere along the way, mankind left Eden and began to use fire on foods. Some people suggest that this was in order to help the food keep longer; others speculate that it was an accident that led to an addiction."[5]

A 2004 article in the *Journal of the American Dietetic Association* says that the concept of raw foodism was introduced in the mid-nineteenth century by Sylvester Graham who "promoted the idea that people would never become ill if they only consumed uncooked foods."[6] In recent years, these diets have become far more common, "as celebrities and high-profile chefs have begun to embrace them, restaurants catering to the raw food diet trend have opened, and numerous raw food cookbooks have been published."[7]

What do raw foodists eat? A raw food diet is filled with lots of fruits and vegetables. It also includes seeds, sea vegetables, sprouts, beans, nuts, and wheatgrass, obtained from sprouted wheatgrass seeds. These all contain the enzymes needed for digestion; the enzymes in seeds and nuts are activated when they are soaked. Raw foodists drink purified or distilled water, freshly made juice, such as freshly squeezed orange juice and coconut juice. Raw milk may be prepared from soaked grains, rice, or ground nuts. Rays from the sun are used to brew naturally fermented or dried tea leaves, herbs, or flowers into tea. Although many raw foodists will only eat raw food, to be considered a true raw foodist, it is generally agreed that at least 75 percent (by weight) of the food intake should be uncooked.

In *Ani's Raw Food Kitchen,* a book published in 2007, executive chef and cofounder of SmartMoney Foods, Ani Phyo presents hundreds of raw food suggestions. Consider the following Banana Raisin Oatmeal for breakfast (four servings):

2 cups oat groats, soaked overnight and rinsed well

3 bananas, chopped

2 tablespoons water

1 cup raisins

Put soaked oats, bananas, and water in the food processor and process until mixed well. Add raisins last and pulse to mix them in.[8]

This Home-Style Minestrone Soup may make a nice lunch (four servings):

1 cup sun-dried tomatoes

2 cups water

3 stalks celery, roughly chopped

2 cloves garlic

$1/4$ to $1/2$ teaspoon cayenne

1 teaspoon sea salt

3 cups tomato, diced

1 zucchini, chopped

1/3 cup basil leaves, chopped

$1/4$ cup oregano leaves

$1/4$ cup extra virgin olive oil

Pinch ground black pepper

Soak sun-dried tomatoes for 10 minutes in 2 cups of water, or until they are soft.

Blend two cups of the soak water from the sun-dried tomatoes with the celery, garlic, cayenne, and sea salt until smooth.

Add fresh tomatoes and soaked sun-dried tomatoes to the blender. Blend on low, leaving a chunky texture.[9]

In addition, how about Mushroom Risotto with White Truffle-Infused Olive Oil for dinner (four servings)?

$1/2$ acorn squash, peeled and cut into 1-inch cubes

2 cups mushrooms, sliced

3 tablespoons Nama Shoyu

2 cloves garlic

1 teaspoon sea salt

1 $1/2$ cups almonds

$3/4$ cup filtered water

1 cup extra virgin olive oil

$1/4$ cup white truffle-infused olive oil

1 scallion, chopped

Place small batches of peeled and cubed squash into your food processor and process into small risotto-size pieces. Put in large mixing bowl and set aside.

Mix mushrooms with Nama Shoyu, and set aside to marinate and soften for at least 5 minutes.

Process garlic and salt into small pieces. Add almonds and process into powder. Add just enough water to make a thick, creamy texture. Add olive oil last to thicken even more. Place in bowl with risotto and mix well. Add marinated mushrooms and mix again. Pour into bowls and drizzle with white truffle-infused olive oil and chopped scallion.[10]

Why would someone choose to follow a raw food diet? Reasons vary from person to person. However, frequently, adhering to such a diet appears to be related to an effort to address a medical problem and/or a desire to lose weight. But there are also many raw foodists with a strong interest in nutrition who hope to maximize their health and/or live a more holistic lifestyle.

In an interview published in 2003 in *Townsend Letter for Doctors and Patients*, David Wolfe, one of the leaders in the world of raw foodists, said that during his childhood he ate everything. Meat, cheese, bread, fast food, and homemade food were all part of his diet. By the age of eighteen, Wolfe could no longer tolerate dairy products, so he stopped consuming them. Almost immediately, he "lost ten pounds, felt lighter, could think clearer, and instantly ended a lifetime of ear trouble."[11]

Soon, Wolfe began a quest to learn more about nutrition. He also started juicing and eating organic foods. Eventually, Wolfe became a vegetarian, and by the time he was twenty-four, he "was on a totally organic, raw-food diet."[12] Wolfe is now devoted to educating others about the importance of proper nutrition, lecturing, writing books, and running a number of raw food-related businesses.

Wolfe notes that the late Dr. Linus Pauling, who was the recipient of two Nobel prizes, believed that all illness was directly related to mineral deficiencies. According to Wolfe, ninety-two minerals, such as calcium, iron, magnesium, zinc, selenium, and manganese, play a role in the health of the body. People who eat an organic, natural, raw plant food diet are able to obtain all these minerals directly from their diet, especially from foods such as wheatgrass juice, blueberries, and sea vegetables. "The most important thing about sea vegetables is that they are mineral-rich, wild foods. They have not been domesticated; they have not been tampered with by human breeding. As a wild food, they are able to survive without human help. Therefore, they possess the strengthening, vital life principle lost in domesticated, 'weak' food.... All wild foods, in fact, possess more minerals than their domesticated counterparts."[13]

It was during an early morning radio interview in 1998 that Matt Amsden heard Wolfe say that eating cooked food could impair one's sex life. Though he was tired from working an overnight shift at a factory, Amsden immediately went to his computer to research raw food. "Something implored me to investigate this right away. It sounded so radical and yet so logical."[14] So Amsden was forever changed. Today, he is a raw food chef who owns RAWvolution, a California-based company that prepares and sends raw food meals throughout the United States.

In his book, *RAWvolution*, which was published in 2006, Amsden notes that he was raised in Ontario, Canada, on a diet that included very little raw food. "Fruit consisted of the occasional spotted banana, a fistful of green grapes, or a soft apple. Even carrot and celery sticks were really just a vehicle for ranch dressing. Like most families, we also had our share of meat, cheese, bread, milk, cookies, cereal, and potato chips."[15]

Amsden writes that eating a raw food diet has transformed his life. "Since 'going raw' ..., my physical energy and stamina have increased. I require less sleep, and can function at an optimal rate for a much longer period of time. I am never ill. I've forgotten what a headache feels like, any wounds heal much more quickly. I am physically stronger, and my reflexes are incredible! Even my vision, hearing, and sense of smell have improved."[16]

Raw food chef and holistic lifestyle advocate, Renée Loux (formerly Renée Loux Underkoffler) is another leader in the raw food field. In her book, *Living Cuisine: The Art and Spirit of Raw Foods*, which was published in 2003, Loux notes that, "Raw foods—or live foods—are whole and unprocessed and make a brilliant prescription for vital health. Cooking and processing deplete food of some of its nutrients."[17] Loux also maintains raw foods contain the enzymes needed to transform food into the energy the body requires. On the other hand, when cooked food, with its diminished level of enzymes, is eaten, the liver must produce the enzymes required for digestion. As a result, "cooked, processed, and flesh foods require more energy from the body to yield less energy for the body."[18]

Loux emphasizes that the most important part of eating is the assimilation of food. "Chewing food well, proper food combinations, maintaining a healthy balance of intestinal flora, and choosing foods suited to individual needs all play an important part of good assimilation and happy digestion."[19]

Although she has been interested in food for most of her life, for close to a decade, Jennifer Cornbleet has been immersed in the world of raw foodism. In fact, she has written books, including *Fundamentals of Raw Living Foods* and *Essentials of Raw Culinary Arts,* and she owns a business, Learn Raw Food.

Cornbleet does not consider raw foodism to be a new concept or particularly unique concept. "Most nutritionists agree that we need to eat more fresh fruits and vegetables. The raw food diet simply suggests that these food should be most of what we eat and should be prepared in a way that maximizes nutrient content."[20]

When developing raw food recipes, Cornbleet redesigns some of her favorite recipes. For example, to replace a standard tuna salad with tuna, onion, celery, parsley, and lemon juice, she created Not Tuna Paté. It also contains onion, celery, parsley, and lemon juice. But, the tuna is replaced with almonds and sunflower seeds.

Cornbleet even offers a substitution for pasta—zucchini. Using a vegetable peeler, zucchini may be cut into long ribbons. The ribbons become "fettuccini," which is then covered with sauce. "Zucchini is a bland and softer vegetable, so when you cut it the right way, it actually has an al dente texture, and it absorbs the flavor of any sauce you serve it with."[21]

What does she say about consuming all those high fat nuts, seeds, and avocadoes? Cornbleet distinguishes between good fats and bad fats. The fats associated with raw foodism are good fats. "True, you don't want to eat too much fat of any kind, but as long as you are getting enough fresh fruits and green leafy vegetables, and not overeating, you don't have to worry about including good fats in your diet."[22]

Unlike some raw foodists, Cornbleet is quite accepting of those who can only include smaller amounts of raw food in their diets. "Eating raw foods doesn't need to be all or nothing.... Eating even 50–75% raw foods can improve health and vitality. The main point is to increase the percentage of fresh fruits and vegetables in the diet."[23]

In an attempt to learn more about the raw food way of life, Suzanne Havala Hobbs, a registered dietician with a doctoral degree, interviewed seventeen raw foodist leaders in the United States. Ranging in age from thirty-one to sixty-nine, eleven were male and six were female. Thirteen had a college education; nine had earned master or doctorate degrees. Four indicated that they belonged to a spiritual or philosophic group. The results were published in 2005 in an article entitled "Attitudes, Practices, and Beliefs of Individuals Consuming a Raw Foods Diet" in *Explore: The Journal of Science and Healing.*

When the raw foodists were asked to describe their diet, twelve said that they ate 85 percent or more raw food. Everyone was a vegetarian; fifteen were vegan. Of the two remaining, one occasionally consumed dairy products, and the other used honey. The raw foodists said that they ate fruits, juices, vegetables, nuts, seeds, and vegetable fats. Generally, they refrained from meat, fish, dairy, eggs, poultry, commercial sweets, and alcohol. "On average, subjects met or exceeded recommended intakes of vegetables, fruits, and fats, and did not meet recommendations for calcium-rich foods, protein-rich foods, and grains."[24]

As for supplements, only one raw foodist took a commercial non-food based supplement of vitamin B12. Six took food-based supplements, and the remainder took no supplements. Because vegan diets tend to place people at risk for vitamin B12 deficiency, these raw foodists are probably at an increased risk for low levels of this vitamin. Among the symptoms associated with vitamin B12 deficiency are paleness, fatigue, shortness of breath, weakness, loss of appetite, diarrhea, numbness and tingling in hands and feet, sore mouth and tongue, and confusion and/or change in mental state.

The raw foodists considered the following factors to be the major advantages of the raw food diet: disease prevention, improved digestion, weight control, and increased energy levels. They believe that food is most beneficial when it comes as close as possible to the living state.

Unfortunately, there is only a relatively modest amount of research on the positive or negative health consequences associated with following a raw food diet. Still, it is useful to review the results of a few of the studies.

A European study, published in 2005 in *The Journal of Nutrition*, investigated the long-term cardiovascular consequences of consuming a diet with a very high intake of raw fruit and vegetables. Specifically, the researchers examined the effect on serum lipids, plasma vitamin B12, folate, and total homocysteine (tHcy) in 94 men and 107 women. It is interesting that the results were both positive and negative. "This study indicates that consumption of a strict raw food diet lowers plasma total cholesterol and triglyceride concentrations [positive outcomes], but also lowers serum HDL cholesterol and increases tHcy concentrations due to vitamin B12 deficiency negative outcomes.[25]

A study published in 2000 also in the *Annals of Nutrition & Metabolism* found that people who follow raw food diets do indeed often have low levels of vitamin B12. The researcher then attempted to determine if this problem could be reduced if raw foodists took sublingual B12, nutritional yeast, or probiotic supplements. Sublingual B12 and nutritional yeast were effective. The researcher advised people on a raw food diet to have their levels of B12 monitored and either consume food with B12 or take sublingual B12 supplements.[26]

A three-month Finnish study published in 2000 in the *Scandinavian Journal of Rheumatology* reviewed the association between consumption of raw vegan diet and the symptoms of fibromyalgia in eighteen patients. A control group of fifteen remained on the omnivorous diet. The people who ate a raw food diet experienced significant improvement in levels of pain, joint stiffness, quality of sleep, health assessment questionnaire, general health questionnaire, and rheumatologist's assessment. Because most of the people were overweight, a "shifting to vegan food caused a significant reduction in body mass index." The researchers concluded that a raw vegan diet "had beneficial effects on fibromyalgia symptoms, at least in the short run."[27]

Commenting on this study in a 2004 article in *Townsend Letter for Doctors and Patients,* Alan R. Gaby, a physician who specializes in nutrition and preventive medicine, noted that there is a good chance that the diet did improve fibromyalgia symptoms—though there is also the possibility of a placebo effect. Moreover, there does appear to be a relationship between fibromyalgia and food allergies, "some of the benefit reported ... may have been due to the avoidance of dairy products, eggs, and other common allergens."[28] In addition, raw foods contain proteolytic enzymes, which have an anti-inflammatory effect.

Another Finish study, published in *Toxicology* in 2000, examined the relationship between consumption of a raw food diet and the symptoms of rheumatoid disorders, specifically fibromyalgia and rheumatoid arthritis. Both groups of patients had an improvement in joint stiffness, pain, and overall health. "In conclusion, the rheumatoid patients subjectively benefited from the vegan diet rich in antioxidants, lactobacilli and fiber, and this was also seen in objective measures."[29]

Under the supervision of two physicians, Gabriel Cousens and Helen Ross, a small but interesting study on reversing diabetes was carried out at the Tree of Life Rejuvenation Center in Arizona. In February 2006 the Center recruited six people with diabetes (two insulin-dependent) who ate the traditional American fast and junk food diet. All of the participants were placed on raw food diets and supplements for two months. However, after two weeks, one of the participants dropped out of the program.

Of the remaining five, all improved—probably a result of weight loss. One person with type 1 diabetes could reduce the insulin intake from seventy units to five units. The other person with type 1 diabetes was completely healed. The blood tests of those with type 2 diabetes were normal. "Succeeding with a group who knew virtually nothing about live foods or the live-food lifestyle, and who had no particular interest in it, was a real test for this program, and it shows its strong effectiveness."[30]

In a study published in 2005 in the *Archives of Internal Medicine,* eighteen volunteers (eleven men and seven females) were placed on a raw food vegetarian diet for a mean duration of 3.6 years. A comparable control group continued to eat a typical American diet. Researchers found that the raw food diet was associated with "low bone mass at clinically important skeletal regions but is without evidence of increased bone turnover or impaired vitamin D status."[31] Commenting on the study, a 2005 article in *IDEA Fitness Journal* noted, "Clearly, more research is needed on the longer-term consequences of a rigid raw-food diet for aging vegetarians. Meanwhile, you might want to consider cooking some of your greens."[32]

A 1999 article in *Caries Research* describes a German study that examined the association between consumption of a raw food diet and dental caries (cavities). Included in the study were 130 subjects whose diets contained more than 95 percent raw food. The control group had seventy-six age- and sex-matched individuals. Researchers found that the people who consumed raw food had significantly more dental erosions. "Only 2.3% of the raw food group (13.2% of the controls) had no erosive defects, whereas 37.2% had at least one tooth with a moderate erosion (55.2% of the controls) and 60.5% had at least one tooth with a severe erosion (31.6% of the controls.)" The researchers concluded that "the raw food diet bears an increased risk of dental erosion compared to conventional nutrition."[33]

In her 2006 book, *Eat Smart Eat Raw*, Kate Wood addresses this problem. She notes that raw foodists frequently have problems with their teeth. Generally, these problems are not caused by fresh fruit. More likely, they are the result of the concentrated sugars in dried fruits and juices. "If you are worried about your teeth, avoid 'grazing' (snacking throughout the day) and clean your teeth half an hour after every meal."[34]

In an article entitled "Healthy Choices on Raw Vegan Diets" that appeared in 2002 in *The Vegan* (a publication of the Vegan Society) Stephen Walsh, who is the nutrition and health spokesperson for the Vegan Society, acknowledged that food processing does destroy some nutrients, but it also inactivates toxins and increases the nutrients in some foods. Walsh wrote that when food is steamed or boiled, only a small number of nutrients, such as folate, are lost. But steaming or boiling enhances the "bioavailability" of carotenoids, such as carrots. And "lycopene, which appears to have profound protective effects on health, is better absorbed from cooked than from raw tomatoes."[35] In addition, Welsh writes, when starchy foods, such as potatoes and grains, are cooked, they contain more energy and their potential toxins are destroyed. "The longest-living population in the world, the Japanese Okinawans, make extensive use of cooked grains, sweet potatoes, vegetables, and soy products and little use of raw fruit. However, there is no large group of long-term raw food vegans to provide a direct comparison."[36]

In the previously noted article in *The Vegan*, Walsh said that one well-recognized side effect of the raw food diet is weight loss. This is because the diet consists of a good deal of low—calorie, high-fiber foods that are quite filling. As a result, the Vegan Society recommends a diet that includes no more than 80 percent raw foods. Vitamin B12 obtained from fortified foods or a B12 supplement should also be part of the diet.[37]

An Italian study published in 2008 in the *Journal of Agricultural and Food Chemistry* attempted to determine the impact of boiling, steaming, and frying on the nutritional content of carrots, zucchini, and broccoli. The researchers found that the nutritional content of the vegetables was better maintained when they were boiled or steamed. Nutrients were lost when the vegetables were fried. When broccoli was steamed, there was an increase in the amount of glucosinolates, which are believed to fight cancer. Researchers speculated that it may eventually be possible to select the best cooking method for each type of vegetable.[38]

A 2004 article in *The* (London) *Independent* contains comments on raw food from Sarah Schenker of the British Nutrition Foundation. "Eating only raw food can limit the variety of foods you consume, which could lead to an imbalance of nutrients. For example, starchy carbohydrates, such as rice, pasta, bread and potatoes, provide insoluble fiber, as opposed to the soluble fiber provided by fruit and vegetables; plus B vitamins, such as the thiamine and riboflavin needed for metabolic pathways, may be lacking."[39]

But, according to Steve Meyerowitz, an expert in sprouts and wheatgrass, when sprouts and wheatgrass, which he terms "superfoods," are included in the diet, they prevent any nutrient shortfalls. Sprouts contain proteins, vitamins, minerals, and other necessary nutrients in their elemental forms, which make them readily digestible. Wheatgrass contains a host of different vitamins, as well as enzymes and amino acids; it "is like a single complete supplement."[40]

In a 2008 article in *Natural Health*, Brian Clement, the codirector of the Hippocrates Health Institute in West Palm Beach, Florida, notes that "drinking two ounces of wheatgrass is like consuming three and a half pounds of vegetables." Clement, who has a doctoral degree, drinks four ounces each day.[41]

Joe Schwarcz, who also has a doctoral degree and serves as director of McGill University's Office for Science and Society, notes in a 2004 article in *Canadian Chemical News* that the live enzyme theories associated with raw food are ridiculous. According to Schwarcz, the enzymes were never alive. Enzymes are proteins that are broken down during digestion. "Many promoters of 'live food' diets emphasize that the 'living enzymes' in fresh fruits and vegetables help digestion and spare the body's enzyme supply from being wasted on digestion. The spared enzymes are then said to be free to take part in metabolism and disease fighting. Nonsense. Metabolic enzymes have nothing to do with digestive enzymes."[42]

At the same time, Schwarcz would like to "go on record" that he advises people to eat a diet filled with live foods. "The fruits and vegetables that make up such a diet contain all sorts of substances that enhance health. But enzymes are not among them."[43]

In his 2003 book *Eat to Live,* Joel Fuhrman, a board-certified family physician who specializes in preventing and reversing disease through nutritional and natural methods, also stresses the importance of raw fruits and vegetables. They "offer the most powerful protection against disease...." Fuhrman advises his patients "to eat huge salads and at least four fresh fruits per day."[44] To Fuhrman, "fruits and vegetables are the two foods with the best correlation with longevity in humans. Not whole-wheat bread, not bran, not even a vegetarian diet shows as powerful a correlation as a high level of fresh fruit and raw green salad consumption."[45]

However one approaches the raw food diet, it is important not to let it become an obsession. In his book, *Health Food Junkies,* which was published in 2000, physician Steven Bratman writes about people who become fixated on eating a healthy diet, a medical problem he called orthorexia nervosa. "I know this disease well," he writes, "because for many years I was one of the most extreme health-food fanatics you can imagine. In fact, I've come to think of it as a true eating disorder, not as life-threatening as bulimia and anorexia nervosa, but definitely in the same family."[46] Still, in a 2005 article in the *Journal of the American Dietetic Association,* Bratman recalls that he "was in contact with one woman whose strict diet eventually led to starvation-induced heart failure and subsequent death."[47]

Over time, Bratman notes in his book, the person with orthorexia nervosa spends his or her days planning, purchasing, preparing, and eating. "If you had a window into her inner life, you'd see little else but self-condemnation for lapses, self-praise for success, strict self-control to resist temptation, and conceited superiority over anyone who indulges in impure dietary habits."[48]

Of course, Bratman advises people to eat a healthful diet. But it is important that the diet not become an obsession. "You can throw away your life by trying to save it."[49]

CONCLUSIONS

People who follow a raw food diet believe that cooking food harms the nutrients. They contend that eating cooked food is far less supportive of good health than eating raw food. On the other hand, people who are opposed to a raw food diet maintain that eating only raw foods is silly and outlandish. More importantly, it lacks sufficient vitamins and minerals for proper health. Yet, raw foodists tend to be slender and generally quite healthy. Clearly, most people in the United States, where about two-thirds of the population is either overweight or obese, should be eating increased amounts of fresh fruits and vegetables and healthier fats, such as those contained in nuts. Hopefully, in the future, there will be additional research on raw foods. Such research may help to clarify the controversy that surrounds the raw food diet.

TOPICS FOR DISCUSSION

1. Have you ever considered following a raw food diet? Why or why not?
2. What percentage of your diet is raw? Do you think you should be eating more raw foods? Why or why not?
3. About how much of your diet consists of fruits and vegetables? Think of ways you could change your diet to eat more?
4. Do you think raw food diets include all the nutrients people need? Why or why not?
5. List ten raw foods that you may try to add to your diet. Discuss why you selected them.

NOTES

1. Mary Spicuzza, "Are Raw-Food Diets Enlightened or Inane?" *The Seattle Times* (December 8, 2003) *The Seattle Times* website, http://www.seattletimes. com.

2. Eleesse Cunningham, "What Is a Raw Diet and Are There Any Risks or Benefits Associated with It?" *Journal of the American Dietetic Association* (October 2004) 104: 1623.

3. Brigitte Mars, *Rawsome!* Laguna Beach, California: Basic Health Publications, 2004.

4. Sarah Merson, "Living Life in the Raw," *The* (London) *Independent* (June 14, 2004) NA.

5. Jeremy Safron, *The Raw Foods Resource Guide* (Berkeley, California: Celestial Arts, 2005) 1.

6. Eleese Cunningham, "What Is a Raw Foods Diet and Are There Any Risks or Benefits Associated with It?" 1623.

7. Eleese Cunningham, "What Is a Raw Foods Diet and Are There Any Risks or Benefits Associated with It?" 1623.

8. Ani Phyo, *Ani's Raw Food Kitchen* (New York: Marlowe & Company, 2007) 69.

9. Ani Phyo, *Ani's Raw Food Kitchen*, 125.

10. Ani Phyo, *Ani's Raw Food Kitchen*, 188.

11. Gina L. Nick, "Consuming Whole Foods in their Raw, Uncooked State: A Personal Interview with Raw Food Nutrition Expert, David Wolfe." *Townsend Letter for Doctors and Patients* (July 2003) 50–52.

12. Gina L. Nick, "Consuming Whole Foods in their Raw, Uncooked State: A Personal Interview with Raw Food Nutrition Expert, David Wolfe."

13. Gina L. Nick, "Consuming Whole Foods in their Raw, Uncooked State: A Personal Interview with Raw Food Nutrition Expert, David Wolfe."

14. Matt Amsden, *RAWvolution* (New York: Regan, 2006) 4.

15. Matt Amsden, *RAWvolution*, 2–3.

16. Matt Amsden, *RAWvolution*, 12–13.

17. Renée Loux Underkoffler, *Living Cuisine: The Art and Spirit of Raw Foods* (New York: Avery, 2003) 9.

18. Renée Loux Underkoffler, *Living Cuisine: The Art and Spirit of Raw Foods*, 10.

19. Renée Loux Underkoffler, *Living Cuisine: The Art and Spirit of Raw Foods*, 10.

20. Learn Raw Food website, http://www.learnrawfood.com.

21. Learn Raw Food website.

22. Learn Raw Food website.

23. Learn Raw Food website.

24. Suzanne Havala Hobbs, "Attitudes, Practices, and Beliefs of Individuals Consuming a Raw Foods Diet," *Explore: The Journal of Science and Healing* (July 2005) 1: 272–7.

25. Corinna Korbnick, Ada L Garcia, Pieter C. Dagnelie, Carola Strassner, Jan Lindemans, Norbert Katz, Claus Leitzmann, and Ingrid Hoffmann, "Long-Term Consumption of a Raw Food Diet Is Associated with Favorable Serum LDL Cholesterol and Triglycerides But Also with Elevated Plasma Homocysteine and Low Serum HDL Cholesterol in Humans," *The Journal of Nutrition* (October 2005) 135: 2372–8.

26. Michael S. Donaldson, "Metabolic Vitamin B12 Status on a Mostly Raw Vegan Diet with Follow-Up Using Tablets, Nutritional Yeast, or Probiotic Supplements," *Annals of Nutrition & Metabolism* (September—December 2000) 44: 229–34.

27. K. Kaartinen, K. Lammi, M. Hypen, M. Nenonen, O. Hänninen, A.-L. Rauma, "Vegan Diet Alleviates Fibromyalgia Symptoms," *Scandinavian Journal of Rheumatology* (October 2000) 29: 308–13.

28. Alan R. Gaby, "Raw Food, Vegan Diet Effective Against Fibromyalgia," *Townsend Letter for Doctors and Patients* (February—March 2004) 28: 247–248.

29. O. Hänninen, K. Kaartinen, A.-L. Rauma, M. Nenonen, R. Törrönen, S. Häkkinen, H. Adlercreutz, and J. Laakso, "Antioxidants in Vegan Diet and Rheumatic Disorders," *Toxicology* (November 2000) 155: 45–53.

30. Tree of Life Rejuvenation Center website, http://www.treeoflife.nu.

31. Luigi Fontana, Jennifer L. Shaw, John O. Holloszy, Dennis T. Villareal, "Low Bone Mass in Subjects on a Long-Term Raw Vegetarian Diet," *Archives of Internal Medicine* (March 28, 2005) 165(6): 684–689.

32. Diane Lofshult, "Raw-Veggie Diet Rubs Bones the Wrong Way," *IDEA Fitness Journal* (October 2005) 2(9): 77.

33. C. Ganss, M. Schlechtriemen, and J. Klimek, "Dental Erosions in Subjects Living on a Raw Food Diet," *Caries Research* (January—February 1999) 33: 74–80.

34. Kate Wood, *Eat Smart Eat Raw* (Garden City Park, New York: Square One Publishers, 2006) 3.

35. Stephen Walsh, "Healthy Choices on Raw Vegan Diets," The Vegan Society website, http://www.vegansociety.com.

36. Stephen Walsh, "Healthy Choices on Raw Vegan Diets."

37. Stephen Walsh, "Healthy Choices on Raw Vegan Diets."

38. Christina Miglio, Emma Chiavaro, Attilio Visconti, Vincenzo Fogliano, and Nicoletta Pellegrini," "Effects of Different Cooking Methods on Nutritional and Physiochemical Characteristics of Selected Vegetables," *Journal of Agricultural and Food Chemistry* (January 9, 2008) 56: 139–47.

39. Sarah Merson, "Living Life in the Raw." NA.

40. Sarah Merson, "Living Life in the Raw," NA.

41. Marisa Belger, "Super Grass," *Natural Health* (February 2008): 87–89.

42. Joe Schwarcz, "Wanted: Enzymes—Dead or Alive?" *Canadian Chemical News* (March 2004) 56: 7.

43. Joe Schwarcz, "Wanted: Enzymes—Dead or Alive?" 7.

44. Joel Fuhrman, *Eat to Live* (Boston and New York: Little Brown and Company, 2003) 43.

45. Joel Fuhrman, *Eat to Live*, 74.

46. Steven Bratman, *Health Food Junkies* (New York: Broadway Books, 2000) 8.

47. Jennifer Mathieu, "What Is Orthorexia?" *Journal of the American Dietetic Association* (October 2005) 105: 1510.

48. Steven Bratman, *Health Food Junkies*, 10.

49. Steven Bratman, *Health Food Junkies*, 19.

REFERENCES AND RESOURCES

Books

Amsden, Matt. *RAWvolution*. New York: Regan, 2006.

Bratman, Steven. *Health Food Junkies*. New York: Broadway Books, 2000.

Cousens, Gabriel. *Rainbow Green Live-Food Cuisine*. Berkeley, California: North Atlantic Books, 2003.

Fuhrman, Joel. *Eat to Live*. Boston and New York: Little Brown and Company, 2003.

Mars, Brigitte. *Rawsome!* Laguna Beach, California: Basic Health Publications, 2004.

Phyo, Ani. *Ani's Raw Food Kitchen*. New York: Marlowe & Company, 2007.

Safron, Jeremy. *The Raw Food Resources Guide*. Berkeley, California: Celestial Arts, 2005.

Underkoffler, Renée Loux. *Living Cuisine: The Art and Spirit of Raw Foods*, New York: Avery, 2003.

Wood, Kate. *Eat Smart Eat Raw*. Garden City Park, New York: Square One Publishers, 2006.

Magazines, Journals, and Newspapers

Adimando, Stacy. "Model of Health." *Natural Health* (February 2008) 15–16.

Belger, Marisa. "Super Grass." *Natural Health* (February 2008): 87–9.

Berkoff, Nancy. "Feeding in the Raw: Raw Food—Vegan by Definition—Takes the No-Meat Menu to New Heights. Are You Prepared to Make the Climb?" *Food Service Director* (December 15, 2005) 18: 34.

Cunningham, Eleese. "What Is a Raw Foods Diet and Are There Any Risks or Benefits Associated with It?" *Journal of the American Dietetic Association* (October 2004) 104: 1623.

Donaldson, Michael S. "Metabolic Vitamin B12 Status on a Mostly Raw Vegan Diet with Follow-Up Using Tablets, Nutritional Yeast, or Probiotic Supplements." *Annals of Nutrition & Metabolism* (September—December 2000) 44: 229–34.

Drapkin, Jennifer. "The Raw Rage." *Psychology Today* (July-August 2005) 38: 20.

Fontana, Luigi, Jennifer L. Shaw, John O. Holloszy, Dennis T. Villareal. "Low Bone Mass in Subjects on a Long-Term Vegetarian Diet." *Archives of Internal Medicine* (March 28, 2005) 165: 684–9.

Gaby, Alan R. "Raw Food, Vegan Diet Effective Against Fibromyalgia." *Townsend Letter for Doctors and Patients* (February—March 2004) 28: 247–248.

Ganss, C., M. Schlechtriemen, and J. Klimek. "Dental Erosions in Subjects Living on a Raw Food Diet." *Caries Research* (January—February 1999) 33: 74–80.

Hänninen, O., K. Kaartinen, A.-L. Rauma, M. Nenonen, R. Törrönen, S. Häkkinen, H. Adlercreutz, and J. Laakso. "Antioxidants In Vegan Diet and Rheumatic Disorders." *Toxicology* (November 2000) 155:45–53.

Hobbs, Suzanne Havala. "Attitudes, Practices, and Beliefs of Individuals Consuming a Raw Foods Diet." *Explore: The Journal of Science and Healing* (July 2005) 1: 272–7.

Kaartinen, K., K. Lammi, M. Hypen, M. Nenonen, O. Hänninen, and A.-L. Rauma. "Vegan Diet Alleviates Fibromyalgia Symptoms." *Scandinavian Journal of Rheumatology* (October 2000) 29: 308–313.

Koebnick, Corinna, Ada L. Garcia, Pieter C. Dagnelie, Carola Strassner, Jan Lindemans, Norbert Katz, Claus Leitzmann, and Ingrid Hoffmann. "Long-Term Consumption of a Raw Food Diet is Associated with Favorable Serum LDL Cholesterol and Triglycerides but Also with Elevated Plasma Homocysteine and Low Serum HDL Cholesterol in Humans." *The Journal of Nutrition* (October 2005) 135: 2372–8.

Lofshult, Diane. "Raw-Veggie Diet Rugs Bones the Wrong Way." *IDEA Fitness Journal* (October 2005) 2: 77.

Mathieu, Jennifer. "What Is Orthorexia?" *Journal of the American Dietetic Association* (October 2005) 105: 1510–2.

Mazori, Daniel. "Raw Reversal." *Natural Health* (November 2007) 37: 20.

Merson, Sarah. "Living Life in the Raw." *The (London) Independent* (June 14, 2004) NA.

Miglio, Christina, Emma Chiavaro, Attilio Visconti, Vincenzo Fogliano, and Nicoletta Pellegrini. "Effects of Different Cooking Methods on Nutritional and Physiochemical Characteristics of Selected Vegetables." *Journal of Agricultural and Food Chemistry* (January 9, 2008) 56: 139–47.

Nick, Gina L. "Consuming Whole Foods in Their Raw, Uncooked State: A Personal Interview with Raw Food Nutrition Expert, David Wolfe." *Townsend Letter for Doctors and Patients* (July 2003): 50–2.

Schwarcz, Joe. "Wanted: Enzymes—Dead or Alive." *Canadian Chemical News* (March 2004) 56: 7.

Websites

Learn Raw Food
http://www.learnrawfood.com

The Seattle Times
http://seattletimes.com

The Vegetarian Resource Group
http://www.vrg.org

Tree of Life Rejuvenation Center
http://www.treeoflife.nu

Vegan Society
http://www.vegansociety.com

Chapter 16

Vegetarian and Vegan Diets

Vegetarians consume a plant-based diet, including fruits and vegetables, grains, nuts, seeds, beans, legumes, and peas. They may or may not eat dairy products, eggs, honey, and fish. Vegans eschew all animal products.

Is a vegetarian diet healthier than a diet that includes meat? Many believe that it is. But others contend that a vegetarian diet lacks sufficient vitamins and nutrients. Some advocate a vegetarian diet for other reasons, such as religious beliefs, environment, and animal rights.

For the vast majority of Americans, eating some form of meat is an essential part of the daily diet. Breakfast would not be breakfast without eggs and sausage and bacon. Lunch would be incomplete without a cheeseburger and fries or a turkey club. Dinner is most enjoyable when it includes a medium-rare steak grilled to perfection. To these Americans, it would be unimaginable to have a Thanksgiving without turkey or an Easter celebration without ham or a leg of lamb. In fact, the Economic Research Service of the United States Department of Agriculture states that "in 2005, total meat consumption (red meat, poultry, and fish) amounted to 200 pounds per person, 22 pounds above the level in 1970. Americans consumed, on average, 17 pounds less red meat (mostly less beef) than in 1970, 40 pounds more poultry, and 4 pounds more fish."[1]

People obtain valuable nutrients from meat. According to the George Mateljan Foundation, four ounces of lean beef provides 64.1 percent of the daily protein requirement. Lean beef is also an excellent source of tryptophan and vitamin B12 and a good source of zinc, selenium, phosphorous, iron, and vitamins B2, B3, and B6. Four ounces of broiled lean beef have only 240.41 calories.[2]

In the past, because of its high fat content, some people stayed away from pork. That is no longer true. Pork today is leaner and lower in

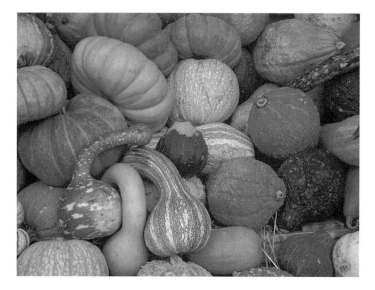

Beautiful and delicious vegetables may encourage vegetarian diets. (Courtesy of Mark A. Goldstein)

fat, calories, and cholesterol than it was decades ago. The American Dietetic Association notes that the following are the leanest cuts of pork: tenderloin, top loin roast, top loin chop, center loin chop, sirloin roast, loin rib chop and shoulder blade steak.[3]

The National Pork Board states that a three-ounce serving of pork contains the following nutrients:

Nutrient	Percentage of Daily Value
Iron	5%
Magnesium	6%
Phosphorus	20%
Zinc	14%
Thiamin	54%
Riboflavin	19%
Niacin	37%
Vitamin B12	8%
Vitamin B6	37%[4]

The George Mateljan Foundation notes that a four-ounce piece of chicken breast provides 67.6 percent of the daily requirement for protein. Chicken is an excellent source for tryptophan, a very good source for vitamin B3, and a good source for selenium, vitamin B6, and phosphorus. Furthermore, a four-ounce piece of roasted chicken breast has only 223.40 calories.[5]

The following table, from the National Chicken Council,[6] shows how the calories and fat content of chicken compared with other animal protein sources (per three-ounce boneless, cooked portion):

Type of Meat	Calories	Total Fat (g)	Saturated Fat(g)	Cholesterol (g)	Protein (mg)
Filet of sole, baked	100	1.5	0.3	60	20
Chicken breast, no skin, baked	120	1.5	0.5	70	24
Chicken, drumstick, no skin, baked	130	4.0	1.0	80	23
Salmon, baked	150	7.0	1.5	55	21
Chicken, breast, with skin, baked	170	7.0	2.0	70	25
Beef sirloin steak, trimmed of visible fat, broiled	170	6.0	2.0	75	26
Chicken, drumstick, with skin, baked	180	9.0	3.0	75	23
Beef tenderloin, trimmed of visible fat, broiled	180	9.0	3.0	70	24

Nevertheless, a growing number of Americans are deciding to eliminate animal products from their diets. According to a 2006 study conducted by Harris Interactive for the Vegetarian Resource Group, "2.3 percent of adults aged 18 years or older say they never eat meat, fish, or fowl, and thus, are vegetarian." In addition, "6.7 percent of the total say they never eat meat."[7] About 1.4 percent avoid all animal products including dairy, eggs, and honey. They are termed vegan (pronounced VEE-gan). There are two vegan subgroups. Fruitarians are vegans who eat only fruit and seeds; raw/living foodists eat at least 75 percent uncooked organic, unprocessed, fruits and vegetables (or fruits and vegetables that have been cooked to no more than 110 degrees). Other types of vegetarians include lacto-ovo vegetarians, who eat dairy and egg products as well as fruits and vegetables; ovo vegetarians, who eat egg products; and lacto vegetarians who eat dairy products. Though many vegetarians do not consider people who eat any form of meat to be vegetarians, pesco-vegetarians are "vegetarians" who eat fish and pollo-vegetarians are "vegetarians" who refrain from eating beef but do eat poultry.

WHY BECOME A VEGETARIAN?

People give many reasons for eliminating animal products from the diet. The Vegetarians Resource Group contends that these include "health, ecological and religious concerns, dislike of meat, compassion for animals, belief in non-violence, and economics. People often become vegetarian for one reason, be it health, religions, or animal rights, and later adopt some of the other reasons as well."[8] And, there is some good evidence that vegetarians are healthier than non-vegetarians, and they tend to live longer. A study published in 2003 in the *American Journal for Clinical Nutrition* entitled "Does Low Meat Consumption Increase Life Expectancy in Humans?" examined whether those who ate meat less than once a week had greater longevity. Researchers concluded that, "Current prospective cohort data from adults in North America and Europe raise the possibility that a lifestyle pattern that includes very low meat intake is associated with greater longevity."[9]

Many contemporary organizations support a vegetarian diet. For example, The Physicians Committee for Responsible Medicine comments "science is also on the side of vegetarianism. Multitudes of studies have demonstrated the remarkable health benefits of a vegetarian diet.... Scientific research shows that health benefits increase as the amount of food from animal sources in the diet decreases, so vegan diets are the healthiest overall."[10]

HISTORY OF VEGETARIANISM

Vegetarianism is not a new concept. It has existed throughout history in cultures around the world. The Vegetarian Society notes that vegetarianism was practiced in ancient Egypt around 3,200 BC. The practice was related to the ancient Egyptian belief in reincarnation or the notion that after death people periodically return to earth in different forms. Based on how they lived in their previous lives, they may be rewarded or punished.[11] A 2007 Hindi Press International article notes that several ancient Eastern religions also supported a vegetarian lifestyle. For example, Jains, or followers of the 2,600-year-old Jainism religion, who are primarily located in India, "refrain from harming even the simplest of life forms." Jains are even told which plants they may consume. Thus, vegetables that are grown in the ground are not permitted "because harvesting them usually means pulling them up by their roots, which destroys the entire plant, as well as all the microorganisms living around the roots."[12]

The same Hindu Press International article explains that Hindu scriptures underscore the importance of nonviolence and following a vegetarian diet. "It is rooted in the spiritual aspiration to maintain a balanced state of mind and body. Hindus also believe that eating meat is not only detrimental to one's spiritual life, but also harmful to one's health and the environment." Meanwhile, Buddhism, still another religion with ancient roots, emphasizes nonviolence and compassion. In the Jataka Tales, which were believed to have been narrated by Buddha, there are stories of reincarnation of animals and humans. "All creatures are divine, and that slaying an animal is as heinous as killing a human." Still, during Buddha's lifetime, meat-eating was common, as was animal sacrifice. However, Buddha asked his followers not to eat meat "if they saw the animal being killed, if they consented to its slaughter, or if they knew the animal was going to be killed for them.[13]

In the West, Pythagoras, a Greek philosopher who lived 2,500 years ago, is frequently referred to as "father of vegetarianism." In fact, until the nineteenth century, people who eliminated meat from their diets were called "Pythagoreans."

Born around 580 BC, Pythagoras was multitalented. In addition to discoveries in mathematics, geometry, and planetary motion and the rotation of the earth around the sun, he founded a society that believed in the transmigration of souls (metempsychosis [after death the body of a human may pass into another species]). To Pythagoras, eating a vegetarian diet was the only way to avoid the potential for eating a former human being. Since Pythagoras, there have been a countless number of vegetarians, including Socrates, Plato, Aristotle, Newton, Leonardo de Vinci, Albert Schweitzer, Albert Einstein, Paul and Linda McCartney, and actors Richard Gere, Tobey Maguire, and Kim Basinger.

Until the twentieth century, only the rich had the wherewithal to eat meat on a regular basis. Simply because they could not afford to eat meat, most of the world's population lived on a vegetarian or near vegetarian diet. At the same time, the European proponents of vegetarianism generally came from the upper crust of society and could easily afford to eat meat.

In 1944 i Donald Watson founded the vegan segment of the vegetarian movement in England. It asked vegetarians to avoid eating any foods of any animal origin (e.g., dairy foods) as well as using animal-based commodities. Thus, it placed a strong emphasis on living by humane principles. During the late 1960s and early 1970s the vegetarian movement gained momentum, especially among counterculture groups that advocated ecology and natural living. In 1971 *Diet for a Small Planet* by Frances Moore Lappé was published. Her arguments for the environment and fighting world hunger attracted many people to vegetarianism. Two more books, *Diet for a New America* (1987) and *May All Be Fed* (1992), both written by John Robbins, discussed the environment, animal rights, world hunger, and the diseases related to an affluent society. In so doing, they galvanized still more support.

EFFECTS OF VEGETARIAN DIETS

Are Vegetarian Diets Always Beneficial?

Do vegetarian diets consistently provide all the essential vitamins and nutrients that people require? First, not all vegetarian diets are low in fat. Whole dairy products, such as cheese, milk, cream, and butter, are high in saturated fat, which may be unhealthful. When consumed frequently, they may negate any of the advantages of a vegetarian diet. Though nuts, seeds, monounsaturated oils, avocadoes, and tofu—foods often eaten on a vegetarian diet—are also higher in fat and calories, they contain healthier fats.

Diseases

Numerous studies have found that a low-fat diet may be useful for people with a number of medical conditions, such as cardiovascular disease, elevated levels of cholesterol, and obesity. In a study reported in 2003 in the *American Journal of Clinical Nutrition*, "Evidence from prospective cohort studies indicates that a high consumption of plant-based foods, such as fruit and vegetables, nuts, and whole grains is associated with a significantly lower risk of coronary artery disease and stroke."[14] Another study, also published in 2003, by Loma Linda researcher Sujatha Rajaram, found some evidence that vegetarians have lower rates of coronary artery disease (also known as ischemic heart disease) than nonvegetarians. "Cross-sectional studies indicate that vegetarians may have lower concentrations of certain markers of hemostatis [blood clotting] compared with nonvegetarians."[15]

In "Type 2 Diabetes and the Vegetarian Diet," an article published in 2003 in the *American Journal of Clinical Nutrition*, researchers reviewed how adhering to a vegetarian diet may affect the heart (cardiac) and vascular problems associated with type 2 diabetes. Their investigation found, "Long-term cohort studies have indicated that whole-grain consumption reduces the risk of both type 2 diabetes and cardiovascular disease. In addition, nuts [e.g., almonds] viscous fibers [e.g., fibers from oats and barley], soy proteins, and plant steroids, which may be part of the vegetarian diet, reduce serum lipids [cholesterol levels]. In combination, these plant food components may have a very significant impact on cardiovascular disease, one of the major complications of diabetes."[16]

Cancer

While most cancer patients are told to eat whatever they wish, Keith Block, director of the Block Center for Integrative Cancer Care in Evanston, Illinois, a true innovator in the field of integrative medicine, believes that is a terrible mistake. He contends that fatty foods support the cancer while starving the patient. Block says that dietary recommendations should be an integral part of cancer treatment. The Center states that "Two decades of study and clinical observation have resulted in the Block Integrative Nutritional Therapy program, based on a personalized semi-vegetarian diet that emphasizes whole grains, vegetables, fruits, legumes, and supplemental botanicals, herbs and vitamins where indicated."[17]

Block became a proponent of integrative medicine and plant-based diets after dealing with his own medical problems. When Block was in his twenties, he suffered from chronic migraines and bleeding ulcers. After conventional medicine failed to solve his health issues, Block turned to complementary therapies, such as acupuncture and meditation, and he began eating a plant-based diet. Very quickly, Block improved.

While chemotherapy and radiation have been known to take a devastating toll on patients, Block has found that his patients manage the treatments with fewer side effects. He is convinced that the phytochemicals in cruciferous vegetables detoxify the blood and flush poisonous residues of drugs and chemotherapy from the body.

POTENTIAL LIMITATIONS OF VEGETARIAN DIET

Not everyone agrees that vegetarian diets are beneficial. Some people maintain that a vegetarian diet has limitations. They usually contend that to meet all the body's requirements, one must consume some form of animal protein. A 2000 article in the *Journal of the American Dietetic Association* described a study of overweight to moderately obese men between the ages of fifty-one and sixty-nine and resistance training. For twelve weeks, nine of the men ate their usual meat-based diet. During the same time period, ten men followed a lacto-ovo-vegetarian diet. The men who ate meat "experienced greater gains in fat-free mass and skeletal muscle in response to resistance training than those who ate a lacto-ovo-vegetarian (LOV) diet."[18] There may be a special concern for women. Women who want to give birth to a son may need to think twice about vegetarianism. That is because researchers at Nottingham University in England determined that mothers-to-be who are vegetarians are more likely than carnivores to give birth to daughters. "In the general British population, boys outnumber girls at birth 106 to 100, but girls outnumbered boys 100 to 81 among babies born to vegetarian moms in the study."[19]

The prime concern appears to be that vegetarian diets may fail to supply sufficient amounts of certain crucial vitamins, such as iron, zinc, and B vitamins. Vegans appear to be at even greater risk. In a 2003 article published in the *American Journal of Clinical Nutrition,* it was noted that, "iron and zinc are the trace minerals of greatest concern when considering the nutritional value of vegetarian diets. With elimination of meat and increased intake of phytate-containing legumes and whole grains, both iron and zinc absorption are reduced from vegetarian, compared with nonvegetarian diets...."[20] Still, there is apparently no evidence that these reductions harm people who live in developed countries. Yet, it is probably a good idea to monitor the intake of calcium in children and women of childbearing age.

Whether vegetarians, especially vegans, consume adequate amounts of calcium is not clear. Some studies indicate that the intake may be too low. But calcium is found in many nondairy foods. The following information, obtained from the U.S. Department of Agriculture, shows the amount of calcium contained in some nondairy products:

The following are dairy sources of calcium:

Food	Calcium (mg)
Plain yogurt, non-fat, 8-ounce container	452
Romano cheese, 1.5 oz	452
Pasteurized process Swiss cheese, 2 oz	438
Plain yogurt, low-fat, 8-ounce container	415
Fruit yogurt, low-fat, 8-ounce container	345
Swiss cheese, 1.5 oz	336
Ricotta cheese, part skim, 1/2 cup	335
Pasteurized process American cheese food, 2 oz.	323
Provolone cheese, 1.5 oz	321
Mozzarella cheese, part-skim, 1.5 oz	311
Cheddar cheese, 1.5 oz	307
Fat-free (skim) milk, 1 cup	306
Muenster cheese, 1.5 oz	305
1% low-fat milk, 1 cup	290
Low-fat chocolate milk (2%), 1 cup	285
2% reduced fat milk, 1 cup	285
Buttermilk, low-fat, 1 cup	284
Chocolate milk, 1 cup	280
Whole milk, 1 cup	276
Yogurt, plain, whole milk, 8-oz. container	275
Fortified ready-to-eat cereal (various), 1 oz	236–1,043
Soy beverage, calcium fortified, 1 cup	368
Sardines. Atlantic, in oil, drained, 3 oz	25
Pink salmon, canned with bones, 3 oz	181
Collards, cooked from frozen, 1/2 cup	178

Food	Calcium (mg)
Molasses, blackstrap, 1 Tbsp	172
Spinach, cooked from frozen, 1/2 cup	146
Soybeans, green, cooked, 1/2 cup	130
Turnip greens, cooked from frozen, 1/2 cup	124

Proper calcium intake is not only a function of consumption. It is also a result of how much calcium is excreted from the body. Some foods have the potential to increase the excretion of calcium. For example, according to the Physicians Committee for Responsible Medicine, people who eat high animal protein diets excrete more calcium. Animal protein tends to "leach calcium from bones."[21]

Furthermore, dietary fiber may bind to calcium and block its absorption. So fiber-rich foods should not be eaten at the same time as calcium rich foods. In addition, to maintain proper levels of calcium, the body also needs vitamin D, potassium, and magnesium.

In "Low Bone Mass in Subjects on a Long-Term Raw Vegetarian Diet," an article that was published in 2005 in the *Archives of Internal Medicine*, researchers studied seven women and eleven men who had been eating a raw food vegetarian diet for one and a half to eleven years. They found that the raw food vegetarian diet "is associated with low bone mass at clinically important skeletal regions." Yet "evidence of increased bone turnover or impaired vitamin D status was not found."[22]

A number of studies have determined that people who eat a plant-based diet are more at risk for vitamin B12 deficiency, which may result in a number of neurological concerns, such as memory problems and the loss of sensation. People who follow vegan diets have an even greater risk of B12 deficiency and, as a result, in most cases, should take B12 supplements.

IS A VEGETARIAN DIET SAFE FOR CHILDREN?

Effects on Children

During the 1990s increasing numbers of health professionals saw the value of vegetarian diets. Shortly before his death in 1998 at the age of ninety-four, Benjamin Spock, probably the best-known pediatrician in the history of the United States, advocated vegetarian diets for children. Apparently, Spock had become a vegetarian in 1991. Spock's wife observed that his change in diet "greatly improved his health and enabled him to complete the revision of his world-famous book [*Dr. Spock's Baby and Child Care*]" [23]

In the seventh edition of *Dr. Spock's Baby and Child Care*, Spock and coauthor Steven J. Parker wrote, "A vegetarian-based diet for children is generally more healthful than a diet containing the cholesterol, saturated fat, and excessive protein found in meat and dairy products." But this type of diet—derived from many leafy green vegetables, fruits, whole grains, and bean products—should not necessarily be low in calories. The authors said that "studies have shown that a well-balanced vegetarian diet has many advantages and does not interfere with a child's growth and development. A reliable vitamin B12 source such as a children's vitamin or cereal or soy milk fortified with B12 is recommended for vegetarians."[24]

The Physicians Committee for Responsible Medicine strongly agrees. "Children raised on fruits, vegetables, whole grains, and legumes grow up to be slimmer and healthier and even live longer than their meat-eating friends. It is much easier to build a nutritious diet from plant foods than from animal products, which contain saturated fat, cholesterol, and other substances that growing children can do without. As for essential nutrients, plant foods are the preferred source because they provide sufficient energy and protein package with other health-promoting nutrients such as fiber, antioxidant vitamins, minerals, and phytochemicals."[25]

An article in 2000 in *Patient Care* said that studies have found that vegetarian and nonvegetarian children grow at about the same rate. "Researchers typically concluded that a vegan or broader vegetarian diet did not impair a child's growth and development if known pitfalls were avoided.... Pitfalls referred to potential inadequacies in calories, protein, vitamins ... calcium, iron and zinc—problems using confined to the vegan diet."[26]

However, others have cautioned against forcing children to follow a strict vegan diet. Lindsay Allen, of U.S. Agriculture Research Service, has stated that, "there is absolutely no question that it's unethical for parents to bring up their children as strict vegans." According to Allen, studies conducted on poor schoolchildren in Africa found that when given small amounts of daily meat, they "grew more and performed better on problem-solving and intelligence tests."[27] But is it fair to compare poor African children with far better fed American children? It should be noted that the study was partially funded by the National Cattleman's Beef Association.

How may problems be avoided? According to Michelle Roberts of the BBC News, extra attention must be devoted to food planning. Without such care, "Food intake may be haphazard, or lack variety, be higher in fat than is desirable, or be short on nutrients or calories." It also may be advisable to be screened for iron-deficiency anemia.

Vitamin C intake should be encouraged. "Foods that contain vitamin C, such as citrus fruits, improve the absorption of nonheme iron [the type of iron in plant foods]."[28]

If dairy products have been eliminated, calcium and vitamin D should be taken in supplemental form. Parents should also be certain that their children consume adequate amounts of vitamin B12 and zinc. The consequences of a B12 deficiency have already been discussed. As for zinc, inadequate amounts may cause "delays in cognitive growth." Furthermore, "poor appetite and slowing of growth are the most evident clinical signs of zinc deficiency in children, particularly during infancy and adolescence."[29]

Adolescents who consider themselves vegetarians have higher rates of eating disorders (anorexia and bulimia). They may diet excessively, binge, vomit intentionally, or use laxatives. Dieting is about twice as common among vegetarians as it is among nonvegetarians. So in some instances, a vegetarian diet may serve as a marker for a potentially life-threatening eating disorder. A study published in 2003 in the *Journal of the American Dietetic Association* noted that "the practice of vegetarianism may be a marker for college female students at risk for weight preoccupation and eating disorder tendencies. Clinicians need to be aware of subpopulations at increased risk for eating disorder tendencies to aid in the early detection of those with true eating disorders."[30]

Toll on The Environment

Although only rarely discussed, livestock have played a significant role in climate change. In a July—August 2008 article in *E Magazine* entitled "The Meat of the Matter," the author explains that the digestive systems of all livestock, but especially cows, produce large amounts of methane gas. This gas plays a significant role in global warming. The article cites a 2006 United Nations report, "Livestock's Long Shadow," which notes that livestock accounts for 18 percent of all greenhouse gas emissions. "That's more than the entire transportation system."[31] Clearly, adhering to a vegetarian/vegan diet reduces global warming.

Religious Beliefs

As has previously been noted, people follow a vegetarian diet for a wide variety of reasons. For some, it is an integral part of their religious beliefs. Many ancient Eastern religions had, and still have, taboos against certain types of foods. Often, that food was meat. Some contemporary religions, such as the Seventh-Day Adventist Church, Buddhism, and Hinduism, promote vegetarian diets. Some Jewish people believe that Judaism supports eliminating meat. In *Judaism and*

Vegetarianism, published in 2001, Richard H. Schwartz said that concern for animals is part of the Jewish belief systems. "The Jewish tradition clearly indicates that we are forbidden to be cruel to animals and that we are to treat them with compassion. These concepts are summarized in the Hebrew phrase *tsa'ar ba'alei chayim,* the biblical mandate not to cause 'pain to any living creature.' This Torah-based teaching is found in all strata of Jewish texts and history and occupies a central placed in Jewish ethical practice. It is part of the Jewish vision of what it means to be a *tzaddik* (righteous individual) and to imitate God's ways."[32]

CONCERN FOR ANIMALS

Animal Rights

Apart from religion, there are many who are simply against killing animals for food or eating animal-based products. When there are so many alternatives, why should animals die—or be forced to live under terrible circumstances—so that humans may eat? Often, these same people are opposed to various aspects of the meat-producing industry.

Though he was the fourth generation of his family to work as a farmer and cattle rancher, Howard F. Lyman no longer eats any meat. In fact, he became president of the International Vegetarian Union. He explained that the rendering industry uses the parts of slaughtered cows not eaten by humans, along with the entire bodies of diseased cows and other farm animals, euthanized pets, animals captured by animal control agencies, and animals killed by motor vehicles. The resulting mixture is ground and cooked. The fatty material floating to the top is refined for use in such products as cosmetics, lubricants, soaps, candles, and waxes. The protein material is dried and pulverized into a brown powder. About one-fourth of it consists of fecal material. This powder is used as an additive to pet food and livestock feed.

In August 1997 the FDA issued a regulation banning the feeding of protein from ruminants (cud-chewing animals) to other ruminants. While cattle no longer eat solid parts of other cattle, sheep, or goats, they still are fed ground-up parts of other animals and fowls, as well as blood and fecal material of their own species and of chickens.

Horrific Living Conditions

Often, the environment in which animals live before they are killed may be far from ideal. *Life Behind Bars,* a 2002 booklet published by Farm Sanctuary in Watkins Glen, New York (an organization that gives sanctuary to hundreds of animals and is dedicated to reducing animal cruelty), notes that conditions for farm animals are frequently inhumane. "Chickens are confined so tightly in tiny wire battery cages that they can barely move, veal calves spend their short lives chained by the neck in crates too small for them to lie down comfortably, and breeding pigs spend years imprisoned in small metal crates, unable even to turn around."[33]

Though public sentiment for the living conditions of farm animals has been growing, *Life Behind Bars* contends that animals lack "basic legal protections." The book describes an instance at the ISE egg factory in New Jersey in which two injured hens are thrown into a trash can filled with dead birds. "ISE was taken to court and its lawyer asserted that it is legally acceptable to discard live birds as if they were manure. When the judge asked, 'Isn't there a big distinction between manure and live animals?' ISE's lawyer responded, 'No, your honor.' The company was found not guilty of animal cruelty."[34]

According to *Life Behind Bars*, "Farm animals, like all animals, have feelings and should be protected from cruelty. Factory farming methods, such as battery cages, veal crates and gestation crates, are inherently cruel, and they should be outlawed in the United States as they have been in other countries."[35]

United Poultry Concerns, a nonprofit organization founded by Karen Davis to raise public awareness about the poultry industry, notes that "in the U.S., each year 9 billion 'broiler' (baby) chickens, both males and females, are raised and killed for food. Worldwide over 50 billion chickens are now being slaughtered every year.... During their 45 days of life, 'broiler' chickens live in filthy litter, unchanged through several flocks of 20,000 or more birds in a single shed. In this atmosphere, excretory ammonia fumes often become so strong that the birds develop a blinding eye disease called 'ammonia burn.'"[36]

In *Making Kind Choices*, which was published in 2005, Ingrid Newkirk, the cofounder of the leading animal rights organization in the world—People for the Ethical Treatment of Animals (PETA)—wrote, "From personal experience, I know how you have to cover your nose and try not to breathe in the laying sheds of the ammonia fumes from accumulated waste of thousands of hens, all kept in constant light to produce an egg every twenty-two hours, assault on your senses. I think of that now any time I smell an egg cooking."[37]

Peter Singer, a philosopher, and Jim Mason, an attorney, describe entering a chicken shed in *The Way We Eat*, which was published in 2006. There is burning of the eyes and lungs that comes from the ammonia. It is "from the bird's droppings, which are simply allowed to pile up on the floor without being cleaned out, not merely during the growing period of each flock, but typically for an entire year, and sometimes for several years. High ammonia levels give the birds chronic respiratory disease, sores on their feet and hocks, and breast blisters. It makes their eyes water, and when it is really bad, many birds go blind. As the birds, bred for extremely rapid growth, get heavier, it hurts them to keep standing up, so they spend much of their time sitting on the excrement-filled litter—hence the breast blisters."[38]

Why are conditions allowed to become so dreadful? According to Singer and Mason, there are no federal laws concerning the welfare of farm animals while they are living on the farm. "Literally, nothing. In the U.S., federal law begins only when animals are transported or arrive at the slaughterhouse. (And even then, there is no law regarding the slaughter of chickens or other birds, who make up 95 percent of all land animals slaughtered in the U.S.) This is not because there is any constitutional barrier to covering the welfare of animals on farms, but simply because Congress has never chosen to enact any such law."[39]

Do turkeys fare any better? Not according to United Poultry Concerns. "Turkeys have been bred to grow so fast and heavy that their bones are too weak to carry the weight. Turkeys frequently suffer from painful lameness so severe they try to walk on their wings to reach food and water.... Turkeys are painfully debeaked and detoed without anesthetic to offset the destructive effects of overcrowding and lack of environmental stimulation."

The situation gets even worse. United Poultry Concerns explains that "between 12 and 26 weeks old turkeys are grabbed and carried upside down by their legs to the transport truck. Jammed in crates they travel without food, water, or weather protection to the slaughterhouse.... At the slaughterhouse, turkeys are torn from the crates and hung by their feet upside down on a movable belt.... They may or may not be 'stunned'— paralyzed while fully conscious—by a handheld electrical stunner, or by having their faces dragged through an electrified waterbath."[40]

One might think that free-range chicken and turkey have better living conditions, but that is not necessarily the case. United Poultry Concerns indicates that the term "free-range" only means that the chickens and turkeys have access to the outdoors. "The yard may be nothing but a mud yard saturated with droppings and intestinal coccidian and other parasites."[41]

When one considers pigs, it is all too easy to recall the lovable Wilbur in E.B. White's *Charlotte's Web*. For the vast majority of pigs, the reality is far different. In *Meat Market*, which was published in 2005, Erik Marcus, an animal agriculture writer and publisher of Vegan.com, notes that though the situation for pigs is not as dire as it is for hens, it is nonetheless far from humane. After industry breeder sows are impregnated at the age of eight months, they spend their pregnancy in "gestation crates." These crates "offer no space for a sow to walk, or even to turn around."[42] Shortly before giving birth, sows are moved into "farrowing crates." "The primary difference between the two units is that farrowing crates have recessed pockets on either side, in which newborn piglets can lie during nursing.... Yet more than 5 percent of piglets are crushed to death while nursing.... Crushing isn't the only hazard confronting piglets: about 3 percent die of diarrhea or starvation."[43]

Why are so many piglets dying? According to Marcus, in the large industrial pig farms there is insufficient supervision. "At Murphy Family Farms, a standardized breeding facility packs in 3600 sows and employs just 15 people [in North Carolina]. Assuming a forty-hour workweek, that means that each sow and her piglets receive barely one minute of human attention per day. That's only enough time to spot the most obvious of problems."[44]

Around the time that the piglets are weaned, they are forced to undergo procedures without anesthetic. "The males are nearly always castrated, since meat from noncastrated males has a pungent odor. For identification purposes, most piglets have deep notches cut into their ears. There are gentler methods for marking pigs, but ear-notching is the fastest and cheapest available method. And since it's legal, the practice is widespread."[45]

Like hens, pigs live in overcrowded settings. As a result, they bite the tails of other pigs. "Rather than solve the problem by giving the animals sufficient room, pig producers resort to tail docking. The little nub of the tail that is left in place after tail docking is extraordinarily sensitive, and even the most depressed and sickly pig will act vigorously to protect it from being bitten."[46]

In *Why Animals Matter*, which was published in 2007, authors Erin E. Williams and Margo DeMello describe how the deplorable conditions also affect the low-paid workers who are forced to inhale high amounts of ammonia and other pollutants. "Workers in slaughterhouses and packing plants suffer some of the highest injury rates among all industries."[47]

Disputing many of the previously noted claims, the American Meat Institute notes that legal requirements and ethical and economic considerations obligate meat packers to handle livestock in the most humane manner possible. The Humane Slaughter Act of 1978 established strict standards for packing plants that are monitored by federal meat inspectors nationwide. They "are present in packing plants during every minute of operation." These inspectors "are empowered to take action in a plant any time they identify a violation of the act."[48] The Humane Slaughter Act requires that

- animals be handled and moved through chutes and pens in ways that do not cause stress;
- livestock must be rendered insensible to pain prior to slaughter (the act details the methods that must be used to stun animals);
- animals must have access to water and those kept longer than 24 hours must have access to feed;

- animals kept in pens overnight must be permitted room to lie down; and
- downers or crippled livestock must not be dragged in the stockyards, crowd pen, or stunning chute.

The American Meat Institute states that the meat industry has taken a number of initiatives to ensure that animals are handled properly. In 1991 it published *Voluntary Handling Guideline for Meat Packers*; in 1997 the industry published Good Management Practice for Animal Handling and the "AMI Audit." During audits, plants measure "livestock vocalizations that may indicate stress, slips and falls that can cause injury, the effectiveness of stunning techniques, and the use of electric prods."

In 1997 the American Meat Institute began sponsoring an annual Animal Care & Handling Conference. Furthermore, in 2002 the Institute's Board of Directors voted "to make animal welfare a non-competitive issue among the Institute's members. Today, members share information that can enhance welfare and welcome each other into plants in an effort to share the best practices."[49]

The American Meat Institute says that the humane treatment of animals results in economic benefits. "When an animal is stressed due to heat, anxiety, rough treatment or environmental factors, the meat that comes from the animal will be of a lesser quality.... These quality defects cause direct economic losses to meat companies." So it is not surprising that data collected since 1996 has found "sustained improvement in livestock handling and stunning."[50]

CONCLUSION

There are many reasons to consider following a vegetarian, or even the more restrictive vegan, diet. For some, it is health. It is becoming increasingly more evident that a vegetarian diet is healthier than a diet filled with fatty animal products. But many follow a vegetarian diet because of religious reasons. Still others find that it exacts a lower toll on the environment. And then there are large numbers who want to prevent as much animal suffering as possible.

Because it is no longer difficult to find vegetarian options on the menus of most mainstream restaurants (or at the very least, options that may be converted to vegetarian meals) or, especially in ethic restaurants, vegetarians generally find it quite easy to maintain their diet both inside and outside their homes.

TOPICS FOR DISCUSSION

1. What are the positive and negative aspects of following a vegetarian diet?
2. Do any of your friends or family members follow a vegetarian diet? If so, have they noticed any improvements in their health?

3. Do you think it is safe for your children to follow a vegan diet? Why or why not?

4. Since reading this chapter, have you reduced your consumption of animal products? Why or why not?

5. Do you believe that the laws governing the treatment of animals on factory farms should be stricter? Why or why not?

NOTES

1. Economic Research Service of the U.S. Department of Agriculture website, http://www.usda.gov.

2. George Mateljan Foundation website, http://whfoods.org.

3. American Dietetic Association website, http://www.eatright.org.

4. National Pork Board website, http://www.porkandhealth.org.

5. George Mateljan Foundation website.

6. National Chicken Council & U.S. Poultry and Egg Association website, http://www.eatchicken.org.

7. The Vegetarian Resource Group website, http://www.vrg.org.

8. The Vegetarian Resource Group website.

9. Pramil N. Singh, Joan Sabaté, and Gary E. Fraser, "Does Low Meat Consumption Increase Life Expectancy in Humans?" *American Journal of Clinical Nutrition* (September 2003) 78: 526S–32S.

10. Physicians Committee for Responsible Medicine website, http://www.pcrm.org.

11. Vegetarian Society website, http://www.vegsoc.org.

12. Hindu Press International website, http://www.hinduismtoday.com.

13. Hindu Press International website.

14. Frank B. Hu, "Plant-based Foods and Prevention of Cardiovascular Disease: An Overview," *American Journal of Clinical Nutrition* (September 2003) 78: 552S–8S.

15. Sujatha Rajaram, "The Effects of Vegetarian Diet, Plant Foods, and Phytochemicals on Hemostasis and Thrombosis," *American Journal of Clinical Nutrition* (September 2003) 78: 559S–69S.

16. David JA Jenkins, Cyril WC Kendall, Augustine Marchie, et al., "Type 2 Diabetes and the Vegetarian Diet," *American Journal of Clinical Nutrition* (September 2003) 78: 626S–32S.

17. Block Center for Integrative Cancer Care website, http://www.blockmd.com.

18. "Omnivorous vs. Vegetarian Diet and Resistance Training-Induced Changes in Body Composition." *Journal of the American Dietetic Association* (May 2000) 100: 596.

19. Lisa McLaughlin, "In Brief: Your Family." *Time* (September 4, 2000) 156: 82.

20. Janet Hunt, "Bioavailability of Iron, Zinc and Other Trace Minerals from Vegetarian Diets," *American Journal of Clinical Nutrition* (September 2003) 78: 633S–9S.

21. Physicians Committee for Responsible Medicine website.

22. Luigi Fontana, Jennifer L. Shew, John O. Holloszy, et al., "Low Bone Mass in Subjects on a Long-Term Raw Vegetarian Diet," *Archives of Internal Medicine* (March 28, 2005) 165: 684–689.

23. Jane E. Brody, "Personal Health: Feeding Children off the Spock Menu," *New York Times* (June 30, 1998) Section F, page 7, column 4.

24. Benjamin Spock and Steven J. Parker, *Dr. Spock's Baby and Child Care,* 7th ed. (New York: Pocket Books, 1998): 342.

25. Physicians Committee for Responsible Medicine website.

26. Lucy H. Labson, Kathryn M. Kolasa, George Poehlman, and Annette I. Peery, "Is a Vegetarian Diet Healthy for Kids?" *Patient Care* (March 15, 2000) 34: 111–128.

27. Michelle Roberts, "Children 'Harmed' By Vegan Diets," BBC News, http://news.bbc.co.uk/1/hi/health/4282257.stm.

28. Michelle Roberts.

29. Michelle Roberts.

30. Sheree A. Klopp, Cynthia J. Heiss, and Heather S. Smith. "Self-Reported Vegetarianism May Be a Marker for College Women at Risk for Disordered Eating." *Journal of the American Dietetic Association* (June 2003) 103: 745–7.

31. Jim Motavalli, "The Meat of the Matter," *E Magazine* (July—August 2008) 19: 27–33.

32. Richard H. Schwartz, *Judaism and Vegetarianism* (New York: Lantern Books, 2003) 15.

33. *Life Behind Bars* (Watkins Glen, New York: Farm Sanctuary: 2002) 2.

34. *Life Behind Bars*, 3.

35. *Life Behind Bars*, 3.

36. United Poultry Concerns website, http://www.upc-online.org.

37. Ingrid Newkirk, *Making Kind Choices* (New York: St. Martin's Griffin, 2005) 113–14.

38. Peter Singer and Jim Mason, *The Way We Eat* (New York and Emmaus, Pennsylvania: Rodale, 2006) 24.

39. Peter Singer and Jim Mason, 45.

40. United Poultry Concerns website.

41. United Poultry Concerns website.

42. Erik Marcus, *Meat Market* (Boston, Massachusetts: Brio Press, 2005) 28.

43. Erik Marcus, 29.

44. Erik Marcus, 29.

45. Erik Marcus, 30.

46. Erik Marcus, 31.

47. Erin E. Williams and Margo DeMello. *Why Animals Matter.* Amherst, New York: Prometheus Books, 2007) 13.

48. American Meat Institute website. In 2005, the American Meat Institute combined the 1991 and 1997 documents into the 2005 Animal Handling and Audit Guide. The document may be downloaded at http://www.meatami.com.

49. American Meat Institute website.

50. American Meat Institute website.

REFERENCES AND RESOURCES

Books

Graimes, Nicola (consultant editor). *Vegan Cooking.* London: Lorenz Books, 2004.

Life Behind Bars. Watkins Glen, New York: Farm Sanctuary: 2002.

Marcus, Erik. *Meat Market.* Boston, Massachusetts: Brio Press, 2005.

Newkirk, Ingrid. *Making Kind Choices.* New York: St. Martin's Griffin, 2005.

Perry, Cheryl L., Leslie A. Lytle, and Teresa G. Jacobs. *The Vegetarian Manifesto.* Philadelphia and London: Running Press, 2004.

Saunders, Kerrie. *The Vegan Diet.* New York: Lantern Books, 2003.

Schwartz, Richard H. *Judaism and Vegetarianism.* New York: Lantern Books, 2001.

Singer, Peter, and Jim Mason. *The Way We Eat.* New York and Emmaus, Pennsylvania: Rodale, 2006.

Spencer, Colin. *Vegetarianism.* New York and London: Four Walls Eight Windows, 2002.

Spock, Benjamin and Steven J. Parker. *Dr. Spock's Baby and Child Care,* 7th ed. New York: Pocket Books, 1998.

Stepaniak, Joanne. *The Vegan Sourcebook.* Los Angeles: Lowell House, 2000.

Williams, Erin E. and Margo DeMello. *Why Animals Matter.* Amherst, New York: Prometheus Books, 2007.

Magazines, Journals, and Newspapers

Brody, Jane E. "Personal Health: Feeding Children off the Spock Menu." *New York Times* (June 30, 1998) Section F, page 7, column 4.

Fontana, Luigi, Jennifer L. Shew, John O. Holloszy, et al. "Low Bone Mass in Subjects on a Long-Term Raw Vegetarian Diet." *Archives of Internal Medicine* (March 28, 2005) 165: 684–9.

Hu, Frank B. "Plant-based Foods and Prevention of Cardiovascular Disease: An Overview." *American Journal of Clinical Nutrition* (September 2003) 78: 552S–8S.

Hunt, Janet. "Bioavailability of Iron, Zinc and Other Trace Minerals from Vegetarian Diets." *American Journal of Clinical Nutrition* (September 2003) 78: 633S–9S.

Jenkins, David JA, Cyril WC Kendall, Augustine Marchie, et al. "Type 2 Diabetes and the Vegetarian Diet." *American Journal of Clinical Nutrition* (September 2003) 78: 626S–32S.

Klopp, Sheree A., Cynthia J. Heiss, and Heather S. Smith. "Self-Reported Vegetarianism May Be a Marker for College Women at Risk for Disordered Eating." *Journal of the American Dietetic Association* (June 2003) 103: 745–7.

Labson, Lucy H., Kathryn M. Kolasa, George Poehlman, and Annette I. Peery. "Is a Vegetarian Diet Healthy for Kids?" *Patient Care* (March 15, 2000) 34: 111–28.

McLaughlin, Lisa. "In Brief: Your Family." *Time* (September 4, 2000) 156: 82.

Mongels, Ann Reed, Virginia Messina, and Vesanto Melina. "Position of the American Dietetic association and Dietitians of Canada: Vegetarian Diets." *Journal of the American Dietetic Association* (June 2003) 103: 748–65.

Motavalli, Jim. "The Meat of the Matter." *E Magazine* (July—August 2008) 19: 27–33.

"Omnivorous vs. Vegetarian Diet and Resistance Training-Induced Changes in Body Composition." *Journal of the American Dietetic Association* (May 2000) 100: 596.

Rajaram, Sujatha. "The Effect of Vegetarian Diet, Plant Foods, and Phytochemicals on Hemostasis and Thrombosis." *American Journal of Clinical Nutrition* (September 2003) 78: 559S–69S.

Rapaport, Amy. "21st Century Medicine Man." *Better Nutrition* (October 2000) 62: S2.

Singh, Pramil N, Joan Sabaté, and Gary E. Fraser. "Does Low Meat Consumption Increase Life Expectancy in Humans?" *American Journal of Clinical Nutrition* (September 2003) 78: 526S–32S.

Roberts, Michelle. "Children 'Harmed' By Vegan Diets," BBC News, http://news.bbc.co.uk/1/hi/health/4282257.stm.

Websites

American Dietetic Association
http://www.eatright.org

American Meat Institute (AMI)
http://www.meatami.com

AMI Foundation
http://amif.org

Block Center for Integrative Cancer Care
http://www.blockmd.com

Farm Sanctuary
http://www.farmsanctuary.org

George Mateljan Foundation
http://www.whfoods.com

Hindu Press International
http://www.hinduismtoday.com

National Cattleman's Beef Association
http://www.beef.org

National Chicken Council & U.S. Poultry and Egg Association
http://www.eatchicken.org

National Pork Board
http://www.porkandhealth.org

People for the Ethical Treatment of Animals (PETA)
http://www.peta.org

Physicians Committee for Responsible Medicine
http://www.pcrm.org

The Vegetarian Resource Group
http://www.vrg.org

United Poultry Concerns, Inc.
http://www.upc-online.org

United States Department of Agriculture
http://www.usda.gov

Vegetarian Society
http://www.vegsoc.org

Index

About the Authors

MYRNA CHANDLER GOLDSTEIN has been a freelance writer and independent scholar for two decades. Her Web site is Doing Good, While Doing Business: Support Socially Responsible Companies (http://www.changethemold.com). She is the author of *Controversies in Food and Nutrition* and *Controversies in the Practice of Medicine*, and the co-author, with Mark A. Goldstein, of *Boys into Men*, with Greenwood Press.

MARK A. GOLDSTEIN, M.D., is Chief, Division of Adolescent and Young Adult Medicine at Massachusetts General Hospital and Chief of Adolescent Programs at Newton Wellesley Hospital. He is the author of *Boys into Men: Staying Healthy through the Teen Years* (Greenwood, 2000), and co-author, with Myrna Chandler Goldstein, of *Controversies in the Practice of Medicine* and of *Controversies in Food and Nutrition*, with Greenwood Press.